To Dennis:

Always remember

" Dogs leave their paw
prints on our hearts forever

All my best

Andy

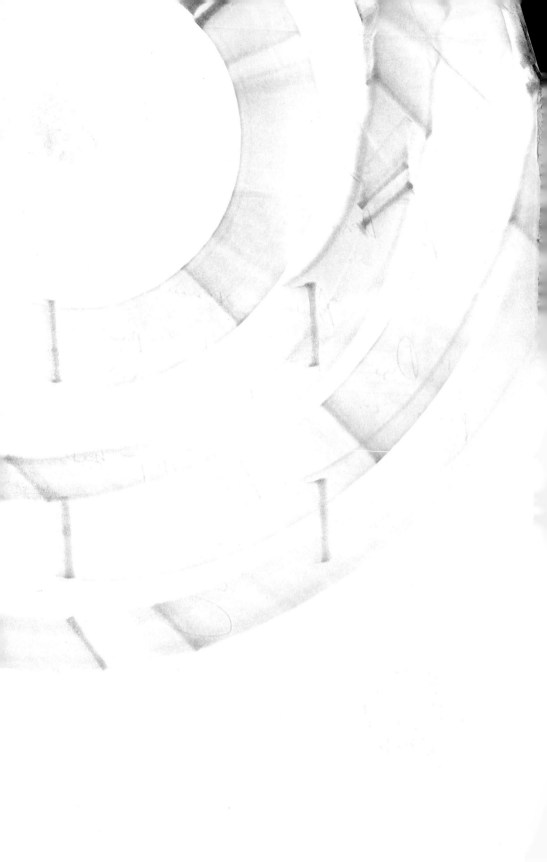

Afternoons with Puppy

New Directions in the Human-Animal Bond
Alan M. Beck, series editor

Afternoons with Puppy

Inspirations from a Therapist and His Animals

Aubrey H. Fine
and
Cynthia J. Eisen

Purdue University Press
West Lafayette, Indiana

Printed in the United States of America.

ISBN 978-1-55753-470-5

Library of Congress Cataloging-in-Publication Data
Fine, Aubrey H.
  Afternoons with Puppy : inspirations from a therapist and his animals /
Aubrey H. Fine and Cynthia J. Eisen.
    p. ; cm. -- (New directions in the human-animal bond)
  Includes index.
  ISBN 978-1-55753-470-5 (alk. paper)
  1. Pets--Therapeutic use. 2. Human-animal relationships. I. Eisen,
Cynthia J., 1953- II. Title. III. Series.
  [DNLM: 1. Bonding, Human-Pet--Personal Narratives. 2. Animals,
Domestic. 3. Child Behavior Disorders--therapy--Personal Narratives.
4. Dogs--psychology. 5. Psychotherapy--methods--Personal Narratives.
WM 460.5.B7 F495a 2008]
  RC489.P47A3587 2008
  616.89'165--dc22
                                                          2007005258

Contents

Dedication

Throughout my life I have been blessed with the support and love of family and friends. Writing this book has given me a greater appreciation of what is important in life. This book is dedicated to all my family and friends who have enriched my life and made it meaningful.

Specifically, to all my family in Montreal—you have made a difference in my early years of life. You inspired and motivated me to reach for my star. I wouldn't be where I am today without all of your support.

To my wife Nya and my boys Sean and Corey, my life would be empty without you. You have blessed my life and made it richer.

Finally, the book is dedicated to all my four-legged and winged family members who have touched my life. Your free spirit and unconditional love has brought true meaning to my existence. You have helped me get a better understanding of what is important in life and showed me how to be more humane. I would especially like to dedicate this book to its namesake, Puppy. I wish I could personally hold and thank my dear furry pal who more than any other animal opened my eyes to the miracles that can be found in the human/animal bond. Thank-you for allowing me to share your life with my family and my patients. Although you are now not physically with me, your spirit and soul are alive within me. Thanks for bringing serendipity, joy and love into my life. You definitely made my "Afternoons" a time I will always cherish. Be at peace my dear friend. You will never be forgotten. I love you!

—AHF

For Giora, my favorite, most cherished reader
and for my three graces,
Gabriella, Sivan, and Talia

—CJE

Acknowledgments

There is no psychiatrist in the world like a puppy licking your face.

—Bern Williams

Afternoons with Puppy celebrates and endorses the power found in therapeutic relationships, and this book represents a compendium of personal insights I've gathered over years. The stories discussed in this book are all true, and the individuals involved have given written permission for us to share their stories with you, but the names have been changed (and often gender and age) to preserve the individuals' anonymity and privacy. The exception is Alexann. Her mother, Wendy Krumm, has given her permission to disclose her daughter's identity in loving memory of Alexann's touching and inspirational story.

Over the course of the past few years we had several individuals involved in helping us research some of the materials incorporated in the book. Ms. Dana O'Callaghan's dedication and sensitivity in gathering some of the research and in interviewing several families throughout the country was invaluable.

Photographers and artists have also made a significant contribution, giving added dimension to the stories. Notably, photographer Tom Zasadzinski at California State Polytechnic University has chronicled my "gang" for many years. The animals are comfortable in Tom's presence, and we are grateful for his contributions and support. Tom's patience and professional manner allowed for the animals' true essence to be captured. We also would like to thank Bill Latham from San Dimas Photography for allowing us to use the picture he took of Puppy several years ago. We also appreciate Mr. Warren Ingalls's willingness to incorporate his three drawings of my canine crew. We believe that his art captured the warmth and soul of the dogs. Finally, we would once again like to thank Wendy Krumm for allowing us to include the photograph Alexann and her good buddy Gleason.

It would be difficult to acknowledge individually all the people who were interviewed and shared their personal accounts of the miracles they witnessed of the human/animal bond. Please note we are grateful for your insights and time. We would like to give a personal thank you to Tamara Ward, Dr. Sam Ross and his associates at Green Chimneys, Carol Rathmann and Barbara Street for their assistance in helping gather some of the information utilized for a few of the stories.

The manuscript was reviewed by several individuals who gave us constructive feedback, and we'd like to acknowledge Dr. Ruth Deich, Joan Hill, Dr. Ron Kotkin, Dr. Jeff Mio, Diana Maberry, Dr. Stephanie Saccoman, and Dr. Dale Salwak for all their help. A special thanks goes to Rudy Gomez for his guidance and support in reading and editing various drafts of the entire manuscript. His insights and counsel were a must! We would also like to thank Carol Kline for her input in the early formation of this manuscript. We are grateful for her insights.

We would like to extend a special word of gratitude to Dr. Alan Beck, the series coordinator for the New Directions in the Human Animal Bond for the Purdue University Press, for his confidence in and encouragement of this project. We would also like to thank Rebecca Corbin, Bryan Shaffer, and Dr. Margaret Hunt at Purdue University Press for all their assistance in getting this manuscript completed.

Finally we would like to thank Dr. Marty Becker for his willingness to write the foreword for this book. You are a true champion for the quality of life for animals. Your insight into the healing power of animals makes your introduction to our book extremely meaningful.

Foreword

Marty Becker, D.V.M.

What a delight it is for me to introduce *Afternoons with Puppy* to you. As a veteran veterinarian and a lifetime pet lover, I have spent countless hours working with animals and their human companions. I have experienced, witnessed and studied the healing powers that are inherent in the bond. As I noted in my book, the *Healing Power of Pets,* "the best medicine may not be found in the medicine cabinet but could be at your side—tail wagging or purring—if you know how to activate it." It is in activating this unique elixir that my hat goes off to Dr. Fine. Not only does he know how to activate the healing power, he knows how to harness its positive energy in tangible ways. I am often asked: What are humans looking for from their pets? Aside from their significant gifts of love, laughter and loyalty, what do animals really offer us? I believe that many of the answers will be found in this wonderfully written book that showcases the human-animal health connection.

It was when I was writing *The Healing Power of Animals* that I became more acquainted with the breadth and depth of Aubrey's understanding about the human/animal bond. Over the years, we have gotten to know each other, and I have developed tremendous respect for his professional contributions. I believe that Aubrey is one of today's most respected trail-blazers and champions in the unique holistic field of Animal Assisted Therapy (AAT). Aubrey is a terrific clinician who has devoted a large part of his life to bettering the lives of his patients. Over the years, he has been recognized by his peers with numerous awards and citations. I was told that he was once called a true Renaissance man by his University President because of the breath and diversity of his skills. He has a strong understanding of how one can utilize animals to enhance lives of people. More so, Aubrey's additional strength is in his ability to translate his clinical insight into every day language that we can all understand and appreciate. We don't just read it, we feel it, we're there.

I remember when Aubrey was considering starting this book; we spoke at length about the concept. Writing a book about his experiences with animals as co-therapists seemed to be a terrific idea. To my knowledge there hasn't been a book written with such insight and in-the-trenches enthusiasm that discusses the discoveries of how a therapist utilizes animal assisted therapies in such a methodic manner. What impressed me the most when I read the materials was hearing Aubrey's passion for this subject and his tremendous clinical savvy. It is evident that Aubrey did not only want to retell his experiences, but he also wanted to weave within his anecdotes the lessons that he learned from his animals. The stories you are about to read will touch your heart. They are powerfully written and allow you to get a glimpse of how specially trained therapy animals can act as catalyst and a means to make a difference. Aubrey masterfully dissects the various cases he sensitively shares and allows you to get a first hand peek of the healing powers of his therapy animals. His stories bring alive the words he writes about, and allows you to personally connect with what he calls his "gang" of co-therapists.

Throughout the book, you will meet Aubrey's co-therapists and meet some of his clients that have been benefited from his technique. You will hear about Puppy, an abused golden retriever, who he adopted, that eventually became his first therapy dog. Puppy, in due course, overcame her fears and made a lasting impression on those she encountered. The day that Aubrey found Puppy was fortunate for both of them. *Afternoons with Puppy* pays tribute to the therapy dog that altered Aubrey's approach to psychotherapy.

You will hear about children such as Sarah who battled depression and anxiety before she met Fine's therapy dog Hart. As you will discover, it was with the support of Hart's blanket of fur that she opened up and made serious life changes. Quoting from the book, Sarah elegantly says, "Hart and you helped me get on the path that opened the world up for me. It is funny, that it was a dog that taught me to talk." When you meet Alexann, you will begin to understand the magical link that can exist between animal and child. Even in Aubrey's own home, the bonds formed between his sons and their pets demonstrate the rapport that can develop and from which both parties can benefit.

Afternoons with Puppy makes it easy for the reader to understand how the inherent powers within pet or therapy animal relationships can be harnessed. But the unique aspect of theses stories is how they remind us of what is important in achieving and maintaining well balanced relationships with anyone in our lives or who we might meet. He breaks down his experiences into to easy to follow lessons we can all practice to enhance not only our day-to-day experiences, but also the way we think about our long-term goals and quality of life.

It is the intuitive power of animals that can help us heal hurts, lessen stress, feel needed, and express our caring side. So sit back and enjoy the read because you'll find enough comfort and inspiration to last a lifetime. After reading this book, you're destined to meet your own pets on a richer, deeper level as you appreciate their unique gifts even more.

—Marty Becker, DVM
Resident veterinarian on Good Morning America
Nationally syndicated pet columnist (Universal Press Syndicate)

Afternoons with Puppy

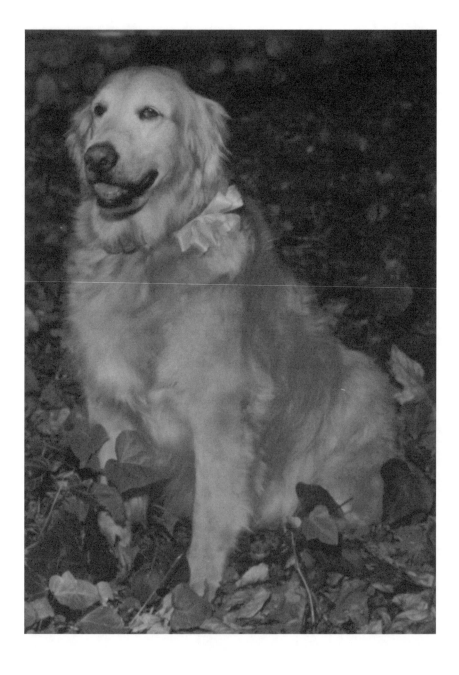

Discoveries

Charles lies on the floor playing with the train set I keep in the waiting room. Puppy is lying on the floor too, in the middle of the train set, the tracks making a circle around her. Every two or three minutes Charles talks to Puppy. "I'm moving the bridge now, Puppy." She responds with an enthusiastic, but gentle wave of her plumy tale. Charles's voice begins to build in volume and excitement. He walks around the tracks holding the train in the air and making louder and louder choo-choo sounds. Suddenly, he stops in mid-choo, kneels in front of Puppy, and he throws his arms around her neck, knocking his glasses half off his face.

Unable to contain himself, Charles sings, "I love you/You love me . . ." As Charles continues singing, his face radiates with happiness. Puppy stands up and gives his cheek a large swipe with her tongue. At this, Charles whoops in surprise and then dissolves into giggles, burying his face in the dog's fur, content and comfortable in Puppy's company.

"All right," I say. "It looks like we're ready to begin our session." It is the start of another afternoon with Puppy and Charles.

This picture of Charles is considerably different from the young boy who entered my office several months earlier. Charles's parents sought help from me because, even though on medication, the five-year-old's episodes of hyperactivity had not diminished. After testing, I diagnosed Charles with ADHD, meaning that his condition was more complex than just being overactive. Charles lacked impulse control and had limited ability to keep focused on any task at hand. In the interview, his mother confided that although Charles could be gentle, more often than not he was in constant motion, moving from toy to toy or place to place, leaving a mess in his wake.

As Charles listened to his parents at our first session, he sat with his head hanging down and shoulders slumped forward, thumping his feet against the couch. His body language told me that he was not only uncomfortable, but also withdrawn, afraid to look at anyone. His slumped shoulders were a clear sign of self-protection and low self-esteem.

For the next three or four weeks I brought Puppy, my golden retriever, into the room with me for the family meeting portion of the sessions. If Charles was moving about the room, Puppy sat by my chair. But if Charles was sitting on the couch, Puppy headed straight for him, placing her head in his lap. By past experience, I knew that Charles sat on the couch when he thought his parents would reveal a troubled week.

I became fascinated by the budding relationship of Puppy and Charles. What was it about Charles that Puppy could sense? What I was able to observe was that when Puppy was near, Charles was more at ease and in control of his excess movements. It was just such questions and observations that have fueled my desire to understand the human/animal bond.

One strategy I use in therapy is empathy, where I attempt to put myself into the child's situation to get a better grasp of how she or he is feeling. In Charles' case I could sense his feeling of humiliation and isolation, especially when he had to listen to his list of shortcomings and failings for the week. But for me to tap into this resource, I need verbal and physical cues such as being able to read his body language. On an occasion such as this, Charles' feelings were revealed in a lowering of his head, a reluctance to make eye contact and a slumping of his shoulders. To lessen his feeling of isolation, I told Charles that he was not alone and, more importantly, that he was a valuable person. Although Puppy may also have been reacting to Charles' body language, I am convinced that she possessed or more readily utilized some innate sense that allowed her to respond to clients faster and on a different level than I could. In fact, I've learned that nonhuman contact allows for a huge increase in a patient's comfort level while in the office. This safe zone is beneficial particularly for new clients since many times it is not appropriate or appreciated for me to make physical contact immediately.

Therefore, in each session, as his parents discussed his behavior, Charles sat stroking Puppy. This need for tactile activity is not uncommon among many of my patients. Several children find it more comfortable to sit on the floor building with the Lego blocks or playing with the train set. However, Charles liked to combine playing on the floor with simultaneously stroking Puppy. It quickly became clear to me that this dejected little boy also needed the tactile comfort of another living being, but one that was neither a parent nor a therapist since this would represent authority, not a peer relationship to help insulate Charles from the adult conversation. Even though weekly reviews revealed occasional setbacks, Charles' physical contact with Puppy gradually brought about a change. When Charles petted her, his posture straightened and from time to time he even lifted his eyes to look at his parents or me.

Several months into treatment, Charles entered the office and, as usual, went to the couch. Also as usual, Puppy padded over to him and placed her head in his lap. This time, however, when his parents left the room for my one-on-one time with their son, Charles began to whisper in Puppy's ear. After a minute, he looked at me.

"It's nice to have someone to talk to," I said. Charles sat, saying nothing, but after another minute he hugged Puppy and said in a small but clear voice, "I told her it's hard to be me."

Even though he and I had talked about ways he could manage his impulses and techniques to improve his attention span, Charles had been extremely hesitant in discussing his feelings. This was the first indication that he was making progress in this area. I encouraged him to tell Puppy more about how he felt, but asked if I could listen. He agreed, and from that session onward I was able to help him work through his feelings and begin to build his self-esteem.

Discovery: Finding the Jewel in the Human/Animal Bond

Charles' story is an example of how therapy animals can help build a relationship between patient and therapist. It may not happen immediately, but I have discovered that the relationship often develops at an earlier stage when animals are present than in conventional treatment. Somehow, animals often offer a more effective gateway into therapy for child and therapist alike.

Surrounded by my dogs, birds, lizards and fish, I feel like a modern-day Dr. Dolittle, although in my case, I don't talk to the animals, I talk with them. Using voice commands and hand signals learned through American Kennel Association (AKA) training, I communicate with my therapy animals so that they, in turn, can help my patients. This method, especially the use of hand signals, enables me to give commands without disrupting a patient. With an unobtrusive flick of my hand, I can send a dog to or from a client. The level of help varies and depends on the needs of each child I see.

For close to thirty years, I have worked, in the company of animals, with children who have special needs. This book documents some of the outcomes I've witnessed while working with these therapy animals. *Afternoons with Puppy* pays tribute to the therapy dog that altered my approach to psychotherapy. Puppy's initial role was simple: make everyone feel comfortable and wanted. But through my experiences with this wonderful, sensitive dog, I learned the deep value of incorporating animals into the fabric of my therapeutic technique. Since becoming a therapist, I have tried numerous approaches and alternatives, some more conventional than others, to reach the hidden inner selves of my clients. Close to twenty years ago I worked with a renowned magician to learn sleight of hand to enhance rapport with my clients, and these skills became popular with all my clients. Where else could they go and see a therapist pull cards out of the air, restore cut-up paper and make items appear or disappear with ease?

Although magic was popular and worked well to relax and transition my patients into a session, I continued my search for other options to make me a better clinician. At the same time, I also wanted to enhance my working atmosphere, making it more engaging and inviting. I wanted people to feel at home and as relaxed as possible. That is when I discovered the power that animals could have on people.

My nonhuman colleagues have the ability to bond with and support my young charges. These animals have been influential in opening doors that appeared shut and providing clients with a blanket of emotional warmth that promotes a strong therapeutic relationship. Although I credit Puppy with having the most profound impact on my skills as a therapist, I have been refining my approach in working with children with special needs since 1973.

When I was an undergraduate in Montreal, I first discovered the therapeutic value of the animal/human bond through introducing a small gerbil by the name of Sasha to a group of children who had learning disabilities, and I think of this as the pivotal point in my discovery of animal assisted therapy. In truth, however, my interest was peaked in 1968 after seeing the movie *Charlie*, the story of a man with a developmental disability whose intelligence is increased through a scientific discovery initially revealed in a genetically altered mouse, named Algernon. This film so fascinated me that I was determined to have a similar pet.

I remember well the day I brought my first mouse home. My excitement made me a bit nervous, and as I was taking her out of the store's box to place her in the cage my mother came into the kitchen. Her sudden entrance and her startled, loud exclamation at seeing a mouse in her home combined with my nerves in handling such a small creation and the result was a small comedy. I dropped the mouse and for the next several minutes chased her in, around, and under the kitchen furniture. On top of this, my mother, now standing on a chair, kept peppering the air with her shock and objections. In the end, I returned the mouse, recognizing that my mother was not yet ready for such a pet. Although I was disappointed, I didn't give up on the idea. In 1973 I finally brought my mother around to the idea, and I purchased Sasha instead of a mouse.

I was so impressed with her gentleness, spunk and response to people that I had her join me in my work with these children. It seemed natural to bring Sasha to the program. I thought the novelty would interest the children, but I didn't have any preconceived ideas on what to expect. But what a remarkable experience my decision made of that morning. Sasha's presence brought a sense of tranquility and calmness to my clients. She was a focal point that riveted the children in working together for a common goal. Over the course of a month, the group built her a small wooden playhouse where she could run around and climb.

I remember one boy who came to group early each week so he could get Sasha's undivided attention. "Aubrey, can I bring in the cage and hold Sasha for a while? She's so cute," bellowed Aaron one day as I entered the building. "Sure, why not?" I replied. My eyes never left him as he carried Sasha in, sat down in the classroom, and let her out of the cage. Suddenly, this ten-year-old hyperactive child was giggling and smiling as Sasha crawled over his legs. Apparently, so as not to frighten her, he sat calmly—something that was hard for him to do. He eventually began to stroke her and tell her how beautiful she was. "You are a real cutey, Sasha. I love you."

At these times, Aaron acted like a different child. She transformed him. Perhaps it was Sasha's size. He moved slowly and talked gently so he wouldn't overpower her. Sasha reciprocated by snuggling and allowing his tender touch. Over the course of the program, I often brought Sasha to Aaron so that he could learn to gauge his own activity level and perhaps be in more control. A dose of holding Sasha appeared to be what he needed to have a calmer and more engaged session.

Over time, I became convinced that there is something special in the animal/human bond. It is ironic that while your eyes are wide open you can miss a great deal of information that might be right in front of you. In my case, this couldn't be closer to the truth. Perhaps it was because I was less experienced then, or the fact that alternative therapy methods were not encouraged. While I was introducing animals into my clinical work both as a student and then as a therapist, I was unaware of others throughout the world that had also discovered the unique impact animals could have on the lives of humans.

When I left Canada in 1977, I didn't have the opportunity to work with animals and people for several years. It wasn't until 1981 that my interest in animal assisted interventions resurfaced with a guinea pig named Houdini. I had just accepted a professorial position at California Polytechnic University and one of the classes I was assigned to teach was in fieldwork experience, training students to work with children of diminished mental capacity. My students were responsible for setting up a social skills and recreational experience for a group of children who came to our campus twice a week. Houdini took on the same role as Sasha. To my surprise, just like years before, the children responded with gentleness and kindness. So many terrific outcomes were initiated as a consequence of having Houdini involved. In fact, one of my students became so convinced of the value of using animals with children that she asked if she could take Houdini with her when she worked at a camp that summer.

This was during the summer of 1983, Laura Jean, otherwise known as Nanny (I called her Nanny because she used to take care of my son while my wife and I worked), was hired at Camp Paivika that is operated by the Crippled Children's Society (currently known as Ability First). The sessions at the camp lasted ten days and served children through adults who have various disabilities. Laura Jean was hired as the camp's activities director, and she wanted to expand the campers' opportunities. Through her college experience in my class, Laura Jean was eager to provide her campers with a similar experience, one where they could connect, care, and interact with a tiny animal on a daily basis. She called me in early July and arrangements were made for Houdini to head off to camp.

I talked with Laura Jean frequently, discussing how Houdini and the campers were getting along. Laura Jean placed her cage by the nature table and at about eye level with the campers. Because of her size, she was small enough to be held in their hands, or for those who did not have enough hand control, to be placed on their laps or held up to their cheeks. Many campers gently stroked Houdini's soft warm fur, or gingerly fed her meals.

I was so intrigued by her reports that I couldn't help making a few visits to see for myself. I remember visiting the camp one day and walking over to the nature center. There was Laura Jean with several campers interacting with "tiny Houdini." One camper, Tom, a young man of eighteen years with severe Cerebral Palsy and confined to a wheelchair, took a personal interest in her. A few days earlier, Tom had agreed to help Laura Jean clean Houdini's cage and check on her at least three times a day. Tom's major job was to make sure that Houdini had enough food, water and, of course, attention. While I was there, I remember seeing the pride on his face as he took care of Houdini's needs. I asked him why he wanted to do this, and he responded in a soft yet proud voice that it felt good to "give of yourself." I left that afternoon, convinced that animals such as Houdini really could make a difference in the lives of many, even in a casual, non-therapeutic setting.

At the end of the summer, Laura Jean returned Houdini and told me more stories of just how special Houdini had become to the campers. In each session it was clear that Houdini had helped at least one camper experience the special bond between an animal and human. Laura Jean related one story about young child named Debi who had sustained a brain injury. As an only child, Debi lived a sheltered life. Although her parents focused on how to help her be successful despite her injury, Debi lacked significant companionship and friendship from non-family members or a pet. Through her camping experience, Debi finally had this much needed opportunity and found great joy in watching Houdini, holding her and touching her soft fur. Of all of the "firsts" Debi experienced that summer, when asked what the highlight of Camp was, a look of joy came to her face and she responded with one word, "Houdini." I was taken aback as Laura Jean told me about the tears of sadness as Debi boarded the bus to leave camp. Along with learning to be more self-sufficient, she realized that not only could she be loved, but that she also had much to offer others, despite her physical condition. She had found a more gentle side to herself and a love for others that she did not know existed within her. All of this occurred because of a tiny animal that made her feel needed and loved.

With these experiences of learning how animals make a difference in the lives of many others, the next logical step was to try working with animals on a full time basis. So when I opened my private practice in 1987, I began to systematically apply my ideas. Over the next several years I added birds, initially starting with a small love bird (Coshi). Shortly after, I added some conures (Tilly, Buddy and Boomer), and eventually I included a cockatiel named Lisa and a small Meyer parrot named Oscar to my growing menagerie. Of course all of these birds came to the office at different time periods over the years. But I was so impressed with how the birds made the children feel that I eventually branched out and, with the help of a few bird behaviorists, I began training Cockatoos. In the next several chapters you will learn the details of how these birds were interwoven into my daily work and brightened the lives of so many of my patients. But my most significant, most rewarding experience, started in 1990 when I rescued dog, whose name became Puppy. She became not only my first therapy dog, but also the matriarch of my practice and was involved in making the difference not only in the lives of many, but also in my life.

Discovery: Learning through Experience

The story of Puppy and my other therapy animals is multi-dimensional. It celebrates the strength found in the animal/human bond and the human victories achieved. But the core of these stories holds another dimension that focuses on my own personal and professional metamorphosis as a result of living with and working among companion animals. They have brought out the best in me, and they have taught me many lessons about others and myself. One of the most profound lessons I've learned for both my professional and personal life is the efficacy of using cooperation instead of coercion. That is, I use positive reinforcement to teach my clients that choices made have consequences rather than using my role as the "adult" to force a child's behavior. My animals have taught me to be calm, gentle, and, ironically, more "human" with others.

In the following case of Diane, it was going to be animal assisted therapy, and especially Puppy, that would be the key to open her door so that she could get the help she needed.

For a long time Diane's parents had told themselves their young daughter was simply extremely shy. But after her first week at kindergarten, the teacher called the parents into school for a conference and told them that Diane needed professional help. In school she was not only unwilling to speak, but also cowered with fright when approached or spoken to and shrunk from being touched. Diane's parents, concerned and upset by this evaluation, tried to work with their daughter to overcome her selective mutism and fear when away from her home. Yet nothing they said or did made any impression on Diane. She refused to talk and at times seemed incapable of speech, as though she physically could not either hear or speak.

My challenge, then, was to break through Diane's fear of strangers and the world beyond her home. The catch, however, was that I myself would be one such stranger in a strange and new place. I first met Diane and her parents on a Friday afternoon, and I had already verified with the family when we made the appointment that Dianne loved dogs, and they felt she would enjoy being in an environment where she would be around a loving "golden."

They are all seated in the waiting room when Puppy and I walk out to greet them. Diane sits with her head down, her eyes directed to a spot on the floor directly in front of her. She makes no move to look up or acknowledge our entrance. Her shoulders are slumped forward and she's bent slightly at the waist as though she's trying to protect herself, or to make herself as small as possible so that she's not seen. Puppy, walking ahead of me, makes a beeline for Diane. Because Diane's head is bowed, Puppy is just three feet away when the girl finally catches sight of her. Startled by the unexpected sight of a large golden retriever, Diane's eyes grow huge and then her mouth curves into a smile. Puppy stops directly in front of Diane and lays her head in the girl's lap. I step into the middle of the room, but signal for Puppy to stay in front of Diane. "Hello. I'm Dr. Fine and this young lady is Puppy." I wait a beat for Diane to speak, but she makes no response, not even an indication that she has even heard me. Instead, like Charles, she begins to pet Puppy's head, running her hands over Puppy's ears, nose and muzzle. She never changes her body posture, but she is smiling and is enjoying her interaction with Puppy. This goes on for several minutes as I speak with Diane's parents. Then an idea hits me.

I turn towards the girl and the dog and speak Puppy's name quietly. When Puppy looks up at me, I give her a hand signal to come toward me and then to continue back into the inner office. Puppy starts walking toward me, but I can tell she is still aware of what is happening behind her because she glances back at Diane. As Puppy walks away, I watch Diane's face fall and her eyes take on a sad and disappointed look. I say, "Oh, I'm sorry. I didn't realize you wanted Puppy to stay with you. All you have to do for her to come back is to say, "Puppy, come.""

Diane's parents stare at me, a look of skepticism on their faces. For a few seconds the air is charged with expectation as Diane debates what to do, her lower lip quivering. Then, in a low voice, she calls, "Puppy, come; please come, Puppy." The parents gape at their daughter, their jaws drop-

ping in surprise. I give Puppy the signal to go and she runs over to Diane, who slides off her chair and hugs Puppy tightly. We watch, her parents in tears, as Diane and Puppy snuggle together.

I know that I have to seize the moment and I send Diane's parents back into the office to wait for me. I join Diane and Puppy on the floor, but at a distance greater than that between Diane and Puppy. I begin to talk to this frightened little girl in a soft voice. I tell her that I know how hard it is for her to talk to people she doesn't know and how happy we are that she has been brave enough to call for Puppy. Hoping to build on this small first step, I ask her what she likes about Puppy. She hesitates a moment and then answers, "That she is soft. That she is funny." As we talk, Puppy sits, leaning against Diane and the little girl's fingers are laced through Puppy's fur.

When it is time for the session to end, I ask Diane to say goodbye to Puppy. She hugs the dog again and says, "Goodbye." Her voice is soft, but it is clear.

———

Diane had made a remarkable breakthrough and could now begin her journey toward interaction with the world outside her home. I stroked Puppy's head gratefully, knowing that without her the session could have gone quite differently.

Over the course of the next five months, Diane, Puppy and I developed a wonderful relationship. Our simple first session eventually changed the lives of Diane and me forever. For Diane, her whole world opened up and she eventually developed the confidence to talk and interact with others, and, in turn, her new confidence rippled throughout the family—they all could now grow and blossom. For myself, I learned to appreciate that a four-legged animal could be a co-therapist. Puppy was able to unlock Diane's silence in a manner that was impossible for me. She was able to nuzzle her and somehow nonverbally reassure her that things were okay.

It seems like only yesterday that Puppy nudged her way into Diane's heart, but it was over sixteen years ago. I seldom get to follow up and see how my patients are doing years after their therapy. A tragedy of my profession is that a therapist rarely gets the chance to witness the gains over the long term. I wonder what Diane's life is like today, and what her life would have been like without meeting Puppy. Would she have eventually worked her through social anxiety and muteness without Puppy's love and nudging? Would another therapist have been able to make similar gains with traditional approaches? I don't know. All I do know is that on one Friday afternoon twelve years ago, a girl opened up and her silence was broken with the help of a canine co-therapist.

Events like the meeting between Puppy and Diane changed the way I work with people in a clinical setting. Prior to having Puppy in my life, I now believe I had only dabbled with animals as therapy colleagues. Puppy was my teacher. Although I recognized that they made a difference, I didn't appreciate just how much they could do. Like other therapists, at first I didn't have the insight or appreciation of the innate power that animals may contribute to a practice until I actually included animals in my office setting.

Discovery: Learning from Others

Many of us recognize the innate benefits of owning an animal, as well as the demands of being a pet owner. Indeed, the two are intertwined and the animal/human bond only works at the optimal level when this fact is recognized. One of the age-old questions asked of an aspiring pet owner is: "Can you take on the responsibility?" Adults can explain the necessity for feeding, grooming and exercising an animal, but do children—however enthusiastically they may shout "yes!"—fully understand? They probably don't—not, at least, until the pet arrives. Even then, if a bond is not forged between the child and animal, chances are good that the responsibility will fall into the lap of the parents. Yet the parent also may not fully understand the potential rewards of the bonding process or the degree to which this bond hinges on responsibility.

For me, the chance to learn about the gift animals can hold for humans came quite late in life. I grew up in a family that didn't keep pets. Although I was curious about animals, they simply were not a part of my family life. In fact, I grew up feeling a little apprehensive around dogs. I realize now that my anxieties towards them stemmed from a lack of exposure rather than from any specific incidents. Who could imagine that, in my young adult years, animals would become such an important aspect of my being? Life is wonderful in its little ironies.

It is funny to think of a grown man begging his wife to get a puppy, but that was me. About twenty-four years ago, as my wife, Nya, and I were leaving the supermarket, I noticed a family standing just outside the door. A handmade sign was propped against a large cardboard box— "Puppies For Sale." I looked inside and saw one adorable big-pawed, floppy-eared golden retriever. My best friend has had goldens for many years, and, being around Carmel (his most recent), I was convinced that having a golden retriever would be a great addition to our family.

On the spot, I fell in love with the puppy, just like a little boy. And like a young child, I began to plead with my wife. "This is great! Can we get him? He's adorable. You know how much we love goldens, especially Carmel. Think of all the fun we will all have." Nya, on the other hand, just like a parent, listed the possible drawbacks. "Is this the right time? Who will care for the puppy? Is Sean old enough to not feel neglected?" He was just two at that time and was in need of a lot of attention. Although she was trying to be objective, eventually her own heart won out. Within half an hour, we had bought our "Goldie," and our lives changed forever.

The desire we have to teach children, and even some adults, about this kind of responsibility is more complex than merely taking care of the body. In caring for this first pet, I made discoveries about life and myself. Within the framework of responsibility for pets are life lessons, and as we bond with and nurture the animal, we also nurture ourselves. This is one reason why animal therapy is an enhancement to my practice.

Children are drawn toward animals for a variety of reasons. When talking informally with pet owners, I hear many comments on the benefits of having pets, ranging from the affection the animals bring to the home, the nonjudgmental acceptance they provide, the love and warmth generated, to the joy and pleasure given. Some adults and children welcome a pet into bed when their sleep is troubled with nightmares. And even members of loving families admit to confiding in the family pet before doing so with the "human" members.

Look at the case of best friends Tamara and Belvedere. Tamara, small for her age and with learning disabilities, routinely came home from school to seek solace first from Belvedere, the family's English springer spaniel. Cynthia recalls, "I knew when Tamara had a bad day. As soon as she'd walk in the door, Tamara would go straight to Belvedere. I'd look out the window and she'd be sitting close to him, both arms thrown around his neck, her head resting next to his with her mouth at his ear. I could never hear what she was saying, but by her facial expressions I could see she was angry or discouraged. I could only imagine what she was saying. "It's awful to feel alone. I try to get noticed, but they just ignore me. They aren't really mean, but they don't care about what I think." Sometimes she would cry. She'd sit this way with him for up to twenty minutes, yet he never moved. I knew she was pouring out her heart, but I never asked what was wrong or what she was saying. I viewed their relationship as I do any other. When she was ready, she'd come to me much calmer and we would talk. I knew it was a beginning and I was happy that she let me in. I often wondered what it would have been like if Belvedere hadn't been around to help her open up and take the initial brunt of her emotions."

Belvedere died three weeks before Tamara was to start her freshman year at college. Tamara gave this simple tribute: "Belvedere was a good dog and a good friend. He never judged me, called me names, or gave advice. He didn't care about the lisp I had or that it took me years to pronounce the letter "r." He just liked hearing my voice, and I was always his first pick when playtime came. He was the greatest! I know I will never have a friend like him again."

What Tamara felt at an early age about the animal/human bond was instinctual. What both she and her sisters knew was that Belvedere was not only a fun family companion, but also a good friend.

I am continually amazed by animals, both in the stories I hear from others and in my own life. Recently a nine-week-old golden retriever puppy became a part of my family's life. We named the puppy Magic, after my love of illusion and sleight of hand. At first, my wife thought we were nuts to adopt Magic, but the puppy was from our friend's litter and once we met her, we simply could not resist. Since she was too young for me to bring to my office, the pup kept Nya company—or, more correctly, very busy. Although Magic's needs were demanding, there was a true joy in watching the two interact. Once again, we had a baby in the house, and Nya's maternal nature was reignited.

Although Nya's love of animals had always been evident in her relationships with our pets, from the start her relationship with Magic was different. Then, just as Magic was due to arrive, Nya was diagnosed with breast cancer. During the following weeks, their relationship was forged deeper and they were inseparable. Before the surgery Magic would snuggle with Nya, resting her head on the breast that had the tumor. Was Magic aware of Nya's illness? We'll never know for sure, but she did seem intuitively aware of my wife's vulnerability. When Nya returned home after surgery, and all through her cancer treatment, Magic was there. Through all of Nya's pain and sadness, Magic was there. She was there through the night as Nya slept, when she felt sick or discouraged, and at times when she was so tired that all she could do was doze in a chair. Magic didn't seem to mind. Her buddy was there and that is what she wanted the most. Ironically, the same held true for Nya. The more Magic surrounded her with love and attention, the more at ease she became. Magic needed Nya and that need seemed to be a healthy distracttion for her. They became inseparable and it was a beautiful sight to see.

It still is amazing to watch the two of them together. Although my wife hesitates to admit it, they are soul mates. I often find the two of them sitting with each other, communicating through words or in silence. One evening, with tears in her eyes, Nya said to me, "I guess we were supposed to get her. Taking care of her is keeping me busy and bringing me joy." These few words have resonated within me, and I'm struck anew by the "magic" of animals.

Mary Hessler-Key states, "When we open our hearts and accept what our companion animals have to teach us, we gain not only the secrets to a more fulfilled life, but also a greater sense of peace and compassion." A companion animal's love for life and for its human companions can inspire us to live each day to the fullest, learn to treat others with kindness, and become sensitive to the challenges others face.

Puppy's Bark Insight: You're Never Too Old for a New Beginning

When I came into Aubrey's life, I was an older dog, who had a very volatile history. Understandably, I was reluctant to trust humans. But my tremendous transformation is indicative of how we should never give up on ourselves or others. The old cliché that "you cannot teach old dogs new tricks" is very misleading. Age, physical ability and circumstances, while often challenging, need not be road blocks to personal growth and living a fulfilled life.

I remember taking hikes with Aubrey where we had to cross over a brook. Initially I was hesitant and afraid of the moving water. Patiently, he waited for me to make a decision of what I wanted do. He knew I was able to jump the brook; I just needed to feel ready. One day, with a bit of coaxing, I risked failure by leaping to the other side. This is what we need to be willing to do. I was willing to take a chance because he showed me love and respect. Consequently this old girl was willing to explore and expand.

I believe that all people thirst for a fulfilled life, we just get to the fountain in different ways. If we respect that thought, we can also recognize there is always room for growth and change. If we want to make a change in our life we must be both willing and open. Many of us say we are

willing and ready for changes but let fear hold us back. A new beginning can be frightening and we may not succeed at first. But the alternative is that we remain in the same place where nothing will change. Each step we take, whether or not we succeed, not only helps build our confidence, but also teaches us more about ourselves and what we really want.

Years ago while Aubrey was producing a film on aging, he met a senior who began working as a magician at the age of seventy-five. As a fellow magician, he was thrilled to watch her entertain a group of second and third graders at a school assembly. She was a natural and had great stage presence. Her magic may have been simple, but she felt like David Copperfield. What an accomplishment for this seventy-five year old "rookie." If she had let fear determine her ability or how far she could go, she would have missed the wonderful experience. Fortunately, she was able to find the magic within herself. We all need to appreciate the magic within us and appreciate that it doesn't matter where we are in our lives. What does matter is that we reach out to life and grab on. Life can be magical; the only limit is our imagination.

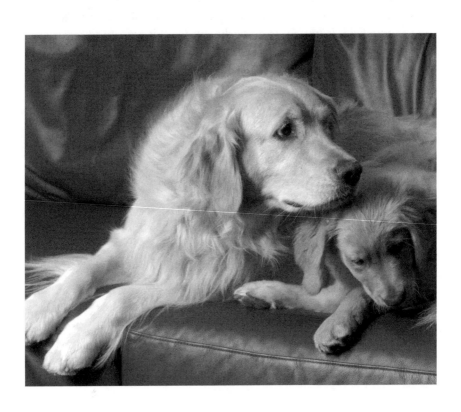

My Life on the "Ranch"

Just Follow the Yellow Brick Road

It is about 6:30 a.m. on a Sunday morning and I am awakened by shuffling noises. My eyes are barely open when I hear the sound of paws tapping on the hardwood flood moving closer to the bed. Hart leans over on my side of the bed and hangs her muzzle just inches from my face and sniffs. She moves down and gently licks my hand, trying to get me moving. I reach over to give her a couple of pats on her head and give her a big kiss on her snout. "Okay girl, just a minute," I say. The commotion continues on the other side of the bed, where Magic is pawing Nya and letting her know she needs to get up, too. Nya rolls over, opens her eyes and with a smile pats Magic and gives her a welcoming "good morning." Magic reciprocates with a few generous licks and continues to prod Nya to get up. As is the case most mornings, Nya beats me out of bed and leads the procession. Once the bedroom door opens, Magic and Hart romp towards the back door. Meanwhile, with all the commotion brewing, I hear PJ beginning to stir, but Shrimp just looks on and is content to rest his old bones as he watches the youngsters harass one another.

PJ decides to crawl off from her comfy pillow, but she only gets to the door before Magic returns and pounces on her. The two begin to tussle playfully—flopping, rolling, and leaping all over the room. I try to maneuver around the two but with little success. Without any warning, both dogs push against my legs and I throw out my arms to keep my balance. "Hey guys, watch out," I say, moving out of the way. "I'm not a bowling pin."

Welcome to my world. It may not be as exotic as Africa, but it is a world uniquely suited to me. Every morning is somewhat different, but rest assured they all start off as hectic. Not only are the dogs ready to get moving, but so are our other animals. As I walk down the hallway, I am greeted with a few caws from Tikvah. Not to be overshadowed by the dogs, our oldest cockatoo lets me know she is ready to get out of her night cage and go outside. "Good morning, Tikvah," she calls to me as she bobs back and forth. "Hi, buddy, are you ready to go?" I ask as I reach into her cage to let her out. She reciprocates with a gentle snuggle before she returns to her excited bobbing and weaving.

Where did this penchant to surround myself with so many animals come from? Was I lost as a child and reared by a friendly, loving gorilla? Perhaps in a dream, but we all know that didn't happen. Nevertheless, where did my affinity for animals actually begin? It goes back a number of years and can best be explained by my recent journey to Africa.

A Trip of a Lifetime

I firmly believe that learning is a life-long experience. It would sadden me to think that after age thirty or so humans stop growing both emotionally and intellectually. I've shared how incorporating animals into my practice has come about. But I'm also pleased to share my latest experience, one that has moved me profoundly because this trip taught me the value of home.

For years my dream vacation was to go to Africa. Ever since I was a little boy, I have been fascinated with exotic animals. During the 1950s and '60s, one of my favorite TV shows was *The Wonderful World of Disney*. It was a Sunday staple in my house. I remember those days well. After dinner we would take our baths and be glued to the TV at 7 p.m. Although I loved the cartoons and some of the comedies, I always looked forward to the weekly programs that focused on animals.

Another staple of the '60s was the half-hour program *Mutual of Omaha's Wild Kingdom*, hosted by Marlin Perkins. Most often, the programs would show some gentle scenes that captivated our hearts. I, like many TV viewers, humanized these animals and saw qualities in them that were similar to us. Then, films like *Born Free* heightened my curiosity about these unique creatures and may have been the genesis for incorporating animals into my life and practice. My sense of awe has never been extinguished and my dream of visiting Africa was always in the back of my mind.

My dream was finally realized during the spring of 2006. After driving everyone in my family crazy and begging them to join me on a safari of discovery, my wife surprised me with a trip to Kenya. Although she seemed excited for me to go, I couldn't generate any interest in her or any family members to join me. I felt like Billy Crystal on his week long dude ranch experience, only this "city slicker" was off to Africa.

I have to confess that prior to leaving I had some reservations about going to Africa. Everyone had a comment. Most weren't helpful. People warned me I wouldn't be safe, and they were concerned about the high crime rate and health issues. Although in the midst of listening to the comments my anxiety rose, my desire to fulfill a life long dream would not be detoured.

I arrived in Nairobi early in the morning, but before leaving on the safari the next day, I went to the Nairobi Giraffe Center and spent some time observing the rare Rothschild Giraffes. Although the center itself has the feel of a zoo, seeing the animals roam freely was a beautiful experience. They are magnificent. A couple of the giraffes walked right up to the platform expecting to be fed, and I couldn't resist. I fed a middle-aged giraffe named Betsy. She walked up to me and stuck her head and tongue out. Once being nudged, I got the idea that she expected me to feed her. I grabbed some food pebbles from a nearby can and began feeding her. I felt like a kid in a candy store. Once I got into the swing of things, I realized that while feeding her the pellets she'd allowed me to stroke her chin and neck. She would be the last animal I would caress with my fingers in Africa. The rest of my embrace would be with my soul.

I was in seventh heaven about my first encounter with the animals in Africa, but it wasn't until I had my first glimpse of herds of animals roaming freely that I got to experience the "real" Africa. From Nairobi, I went to Samburu and the Mara (near the Tanzanian border—the gateway to the Serengeti). Here, I experienced the heart of Kenya. The trip is not a comfortable drive; the roads in Kenya are rustic, and, on my part, there was a lot of bouncing and grabbing on to the car for security.

But I will never forget the emotions that went through me as we drew closer to our first night's lodging in Samburu. On the side of the road were a herd of zebras and wildebeests. My mouth dropped when I first saw them. The City Slicker was really here, in Africa. The zebras were close enough to touch, and, unlike my zoo visits, they were not fenced in. Several of them were frolicking and grazing on the grass. From the corner of my eye I saw a baby zebra that couldn't have been older than a few months. She was running beside her mother and looked so innocent. I just couldn't believe what I was seeing. While the wildebeests seemed content to stay away from the van, I found it fascinating that the animals were so close to the village.

For the next several days I took daily game-drives. I never knew what I'd see. In fact, on a few of the drives we weren't able to find any animals. Although somewhat disappointing, I was expecting that. Animals in the wild rarely stay in any one place for long, and the drivers can only estimate where the animals might roam on any given day.

But I was never disappointed. The landscape was beautiful and when we did sight animals, it was spectacular. Each animal I saw brought out a different emotion. Cheetahs and lions were a couple of my favorites. When I saw my first couple of cheetahs, resting under a tree, I was speechless. Their bodies are masterpieces, and I now understand why they are outstanding runners. Because of this, I got busy snapping pictures before they took flight. One afternoon, after several hours of searching, we saw a large herd of elephants parading to the water. Among the herd was a baby elephant. She was guarded by her mom and needed prodding to follow the herd as they went into the water. But once in the water its joy was evident; like any human baby she splashed and frolicked.

Ironically, although I loved seeing all of the large and exotic animals, my heart was stolen by the smallest members of the gazelle family; an animal called a dick dick. These are very shy and timid creatures. In most cases, they keep their distance from predators and humans alike. Late one afternoon in my campground in the Mara, I spotted a couple of dick dicks wandering around. They didn't seem to startle when they saw me, so I decided to sit on the ground and watch. Luckily, I had my camera and was able to zoom in even closer for a better view. As I watched from a distance, I could see the individual strands in their dark brown fur as they nibbled on the trees. This is what I loved to do the entire trip, just take my time and observe the animals as they went about their daily life.

My only regret about the whole safari is, although you are in the wilderness when out on game drives, you are often surrounded by many other tour vehicles. It's like being in Disneyland. There are crowds at all the major attractions. For example, when I saw my first leopard there were about nine other vehicles circling it. She must have been used to this because she gave us little attention. I was told many of the animals are used to the "white vans" and tend to ignore them. My other major disappointment has more to do with the other visitors. Many of them are more interested in getting the best photo than taking time to enjoy the animals in the wild. I must have heard at least a hundred times, "Oh that is a great shot" or "Just wait, you'll get the shot you want." Too often I felt that I was on a picture safari, running from place to place hunting for the best photo-op rather than experiencing the setting of Africa. I remember seeing a small heard of zebras. I would have loved to just sit and watch for hours, but we didn't even stop. We drove right by them in the quest to find a pride of lions. I asked the guide if we could stop and he told me, "Don't worry, you will see more zebras later." I didn't argue, but I knew I would never be able to capture that specific moment again. A photo shoot in Africa is like shopping in a foreign country. If you see something you like, buy it because you may never see it again. Now I know why a photographer friend of mine warned me, "Always have your camera at the ready. Be paparazzi."

As my trip came to a close, I reflected on what the experience meant to me. Did my visit to Africa help me understand any better my soulful connection to animals? Did seeing all of those beautiful, exotic creatures enable me to understand why I have become so connected to animals? Going to Africa had been my dream for over twenty years, and I will cherish the memories for a lifetime. However, I walked away feeling in a muddle because, although I loved what I had seen, it didn't really help me understand the root of my affection towards animals. In fact, I had begun to miss my own "wild" gang; so, I clicked my heels three times, and before I knew it I was back in California with my loving family.

Like Dorothy in the *Wizard of Oz,* who followed the yellow brick road trying to get back to Kansas, I began to realize that my curiosity of animals may have originated by watching TV shows like *Wild Kingdom* or *Disney's Wonderful World* on Sunday nights, but it is my own group of animals at home that really fascinate me because of the strong connection to them. Sure PJ isn't as majestic as a lioness nor is Shrimp as magnificent as a leopard, but they are mine and I adore them all. As I flew back from Nairobi, I thought of all of them and gained new insight and appreciation for how lucky I am. I really was like Dorothy flying back to Kansas. When I got home I received a king's welcome from the gang. PJ and Magic led the pack and were jumping with excitement. Bringing up the rear were Hart and old Shrimp, letting me know they missed me too. I flew all the way to Africa only to realize it was here that my connection rested. It is home, family, and friends that bring us joy and stability. They enable us to dream, to reach for something new. I learned, just as

Dorothy does, that magic truly only happens in establishing loving and stable relationships. As Dorothy says, "There's no place like home."

A life filled with an animal companion can't get much better. Expect the unexpected and you'll enjoy what you find (at least most of the time). It is hard for me to imagine any other way of life. I just wouldn't be complete without my extended family. For me this morning is just like any other—hectic, noisy, and filled with pleasure.

Introductions seem appropriate right now. They will help you become more familiar with some of the animals before you meet them within the stories. Also, you'll meet several other remarkable animals throughout this book; their stories are equally as important, but they will be introduced as the book unfolds. By the end of this chapter, you'll have a better idea of what living with my menagerie is like. It is not always glamour and fun, but it is always interesting. My animals, like most of us, go to work and there is a conscious effort on my part to make this distinction. While at home our animals are part of the family, and they are well-loved pets. The first animal to win my heart completely was Puppy.

I have to confess, when looking back over those seventeen years, it is relationships such as Puppy and Diane's that changed the way I clinically worked with people. Prior to having Puppy in my life, I was merely dabbling in pairing clients and animals as therapy colleagues. Sure, I recognized they made a difference, but I didn't appreciate how much. Unfortunately, this is a misunderstanding that many therapists develop. They don't have the insight or appreciation of the innate therapeutic power that animals may contribute. Also, they don't possess the awareness of how best to incorporate the animals in a manner that can make the most difference. Some, unfortunately, also don't take into consideration the welfare of the animals. They view the animals as being there at their beck and call. Often the animals' personal interests are not a priority, and, of course, they must be.

Things have changed in my life over the years. Not only am I immersed in having animals as co-therapists, but also I would never jeopardize their physical and/or emotional safety just for the sake of helping my clients. There has to be a balance. They get breaks, walks, treats and lots of attention. I do have to watch that they aren't given too many snacks, so the treats that are given throughout the day are built into their daily diet. Over the years, I have never had a client that treated them poorly, but I have developed guidelines for their safety. The bottom line is that they aren't part of my work as an attraction, but rather as a support network. My animals have opened the eyes of my heart. They have allowed me to see clearer the pain my patients experience and to make the therapeutic bond stronger.

Early Relationships

Although I noted my initial work with people and animals stemmed all the way back to Sasha, I began using birds and fish in 1987 when I started my practice as a psychologist and before I started using dogs. Over the years, I have also added a couple of rabbits as well as small lizards (bearded dragon, anoles and small geckos).

The fish were initially selected to help with the ambience. I always wanted my office to be inviting and comfortable. I believed then, as I do today, that the therapeutic process begins when a person enters the office. Making the atmosphere more pleasant has always been important to me. I believed an aquatic tank or two would have a relaxing effect in the waiting room. How right I was. Not only do the fish generate discussion, but they instill a sense of relaxation. The plants swaying gently, fish gliding, and the soft burble of the water pump often work as a sedative. It isn't uncommon for me to return to the waiting room and find a parent napping. The fish also are a source of conversation. Children are interested in the marine life and ask lots of questions. I now have three large tanks scattered throughout my office. Two are fresh water and the third is a large coral reef, which also has several species of salt water fish.

After seeing the value of the fish, and remembering my days with Sasha, I decided to expand the animal presence in the office. I have always been fascinated with birds; especially those who are hand fed and receptive to human touch. I began with little birds so I could become more confident in interacting with the species. To assure the best choice possible, I spent almost a year talking with various avian specialists before I purchased my first bird. I spoke with people who helped me learn what birds need and how to best train them to interact with people. Throughout the next few chapters, you will hear about many of the birds I work with. You will hear how a few dusky Conures named Tilly, Buddy, Boomer and Polly have impacted the lives of children who were lonely, felt different and even were abused. You will also hear about Coshi, a peach face lovebird who had a tremendous impact on the life of my youngest son, Corey. When Corey was a preschooler, they were literally inseparable. In fact, she was one of his closest playmates, often hanging on his shirt or on his pants as he went around the house.

My first large bird was a bare-eyed cockatoo I named Tikvah, the "bird of hope." The children I work with fell in love with her. Bird experts told me that cockatoos are the best possible choice for therapy birds because they love attention and enjoy interacting with humans. As expected, the young bird Tikvah was very affectionate and animated. She is now sixteen years old and still loves to dance whenever she hears music. Her love of dance started as a young bird as she was establishing a loving relationship with my older son Sean. One of the nightly rituals she enjoyed was helping tuck Sean into bed. When my wife or I went to say goodnight to Sean, Tikvah could be seen waddling down the hallway, ready to say her goodnight as well.

She'd climb up on Sean's bed and give him her undying attention. This usually ended up in Sean humming a few bars of a song, and Tikvah "rocking out" on his bed. Even today, they have a very close relationship. When he comes home from college, she caws for him to pick her up. Once seated together, she still snuggles with her "little" boy, though now he is six feet-five inches tall.

Since then, I have added two other cockatoos to my family of therapy birds. To ensure that they all get the attention they deserve and need, the birds take turns participating in the office work. In 1986, I adopted a sulfur-crested cockatoo that the breeder couldn't sell because another bird had bitten off one of her toes. I named her Starlight, in honor of Andrew Lloyd Weber's play *Starlight Express*. The story revolves around a battered steam engine named Rusty who is encouraged to race a flashy diesel locomotive. Although the odds of winning are minimal, the play represents the triumph of the spirit and the need to never give up. Thus, it was the perfect name for a therapy bird. Over the decade, she has become an inspiration to many children who needed to learn that one can overcome hardships.

Finally in the summer of 1994, I purchased my last cockatoo. She is a sweet umbrella cockatoo named Snowflake. For the first six weeks I hand fed Snow so our bond would grow strong. Umbrellas are bright, but they can be mischievous. One of Snowflake's greatest fetishes is her love of picking the keys off computer keyboards. She really doesn't destroy them, but before I knew how to put all the letters back, I was buying new keyboards almost monthly. Even with all of her idiosyncrasies, Snow is a wonderful bird. She enjoys sitting in on therapy, and she often joins the children and the dogs on our therapy walks, sitting on one of my shoulders.

Finally, there are the dogs. As this book will unfold, a few other dogs will be shown as significant in my afternoons, especially since

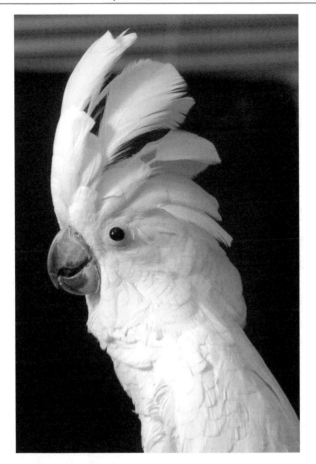

Puppy has, unfortunately, left us.

Puppy: The Afternoon Girl

Puppy's charisma was unfailing. She radiated from within and made our afternoons a time for learning and transformation. Hour by hour she worked her magic and made children and their families comfortable. They were coming to confront difficult issues, but it was made easier by her presence. At times, it merely was an unbridled greeting filled with love; while on other occasions, it was an act of compassion and support that made a difference for a child or her/his family. She brought warmth into a place that could often be perceived as cold, frightening, and uncomfortable.

Puppy came into our lives April of 1990. She had escaped from her previous abusive life with the hope of having a better one, at least a safer one. She was a foundling, a canine Moses, who brought magic to the magician, and I was like the Pharaoh's daughter who found Moses in the bulrushes. There was something mystical about the meeting that brought great changes for everyone who came to know Puppy. When we found her running on the streets near our home, we could see she was an abused and neglected dog. She was scared of human touch and was missing a few of her teeth. It took some time for her to become more at ease with human contact. Nevertheless, over a little time and with kindness, love, and lots of attention, Puppy became more trusting. She and I particularly connected and soon were inseparable. Puppy thrived with the attention; she soon loved being around people.

As she relearned to trust, I hoped she could join me in my work with children. I saw her potential, that her great warmth along with a seasoned maturity could benefit my clients. Puppy had a hard beginning to life, and I felt she could help others understand that life has many turns and that goodness can be achieved even in times of adversity. The more I thought about it, the more I believed Puppy would be a good therapy dog, especially since she had a calming effect on most anyone she encountered. Many people do not to understand a dog's ability to assimilate past experiences and apply them to new encounters. Puppy had that singular ability to sense what people needed and give freely of herself.

This was probably the best decision I ever made. Over the course of a decade, Puppy became the matriarch and ambassador of my office. She loved going to work and my clients loved her. She became my receptionist, always greeting the new arrivals; my office manager, always making sure everyone was where they were supposed to be; and, most importantly, she became my co-therapist, demonstrating sensitivity and compassion. Because of all this, she enhanced my abilities as a therapist.

She had a wonderful air about her. She approached people with grace; her face radiated welcome. She knew how to enter gently into my clients' worlds. She was a pro at reaching out and relating. Puppy became more maternal and seasoned as the years progressed. Like a pitcher who is plucked from the bullpen to finish off a game, Puppy was my "closer." She would either get the patients warmed up to see me, or she would come in at some point and instinctively enhance the relationship between the client and myself. She could relax them and get them to open up; she got them to act more human. Perhaps it was because she glowed from the inside, or perhaps the injustices of her early life made it easier for her to relate to others. In therapist lingo, she knew how to apply unconditional positive regard, a method used by the famous psychotherapist Carl Rogers.

We were a great team. She was Ginger to my Fred, and we danced well with each other. We knew how to make hard moves look easy, and we danced in synchrony. It is hard without her. We were inseparable. Although she passed on in October of 2000, her impact in molding this humanistic therapist is beyond words. She not only blessed my clinical life, but also enriched my family with her gentleness and innate loving nature.

Puppy's Legacy: Shrimp

He was the runt of Puppy's litter and was born in June of 1991, a couple of months after we rescued Puppy. We had gone to the veterinarian earlier that day and he told us that Puppy was ready to give birth at any moment. In fact it didn't take long at all. By the time we got home, she was ready. Throughout the long afternoon Puppy actually delivered twelve puppies. Shrimp's welcome to the world was quite traumatic for him because he was the smallest of the bunch and had the hardest time breathing on his own. I noticed quickly that he was struggling and decided to jump into the car and take him to our veterinarian. After getting him some oxygen to help him breathe, I was informed that he was so tiny that he needed to be tube fed so he could get the sustenance that he needed. I became so enamored with this poor little guy that I committed myself to the frequent feedings. He went wherever I went, including a hockey sports camp where I did motivational talks.

As one can appreciate, once the bond between us began to strengthen, it was very hard to adopt him out with his siblings. Shrimp was the only pup we kept from Puppy's litter, and I never intended for him to become a therapy dog. But when Shrimp was only one month old, I was asked to be the commencement speaker for a graduation ceremony for young adults with mental retardation who had just completed a year-long training program for independent living. Shrimp was the inspiration of my talk. As I stood at the podium, sitting in front of me were twenty young adults whom educators had given up on when they were children. Their lives weren't easy as they struggled to find their niche. However, today marked a new page in their lives. They had learned to be responsible for themselves—to shop, clean, pay bills, and hold down a job. Today was their day.

My way of paying tribute to their accomplishments and to discuss the challenges ahead of them was through Shrimp's story. I even brought some slides of my new young friend and shared his fight to stay alive. More importantly, I talked about the love that we had established. Shrimp didn't need everyone to believe in him. He just needed one person that would give him a chance, and that happened to be me. I didn't care that he was the smallest and weakest; he was a fighter that deserved a chance. These young adults, too, were fighters that deserved every opportunity to be the best they could be—a lesson all of us need to be reminded of from time to time, and Shrimp was the perfect illustration.

Eventually, at the age of eight years, Shrimp became an integral

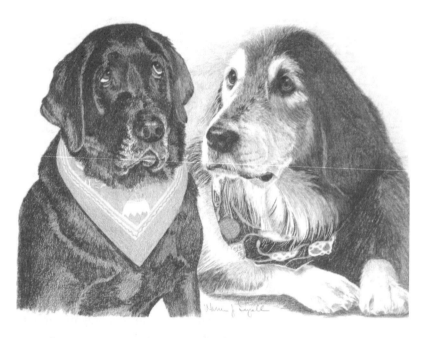

part of my practice. He has aged gracefully and is no longer as active in my practice. His recent claim to fame (as I call it) was an article on senior dogs that appeared in the May 2006 edition of *Dog Fancy* magazine. Shrimp's picture was featured at the top of the article and I couldn't be prouder. I even had copies in the office to show to all of his fans. Shrimp was now a Dog Playmate of the Month. Seriously, the title of the column was called *"Try a Little Tenderness,"* a title that actually got its name from a quote I shared in an interview with the magazine. I was being interviewed about why and how we need to love our older dogs. I remember telling the writer how important it was for me to give Shrimp the best I could, especially as he was aging.

Hart

While Corey (my youngest son) and I were in Geneva, Switzerland in 1994 attending a conference on human-animal interactions, he fell in love with a black lab guide dog giving demonstrations. Corey came back home wanting to raise a guide dog, and in 1997, he became a puppy raiser for Guide Dogs of America. My grandfather was blind, and in some ways preparing a dog to assist the blind was done in tribute him.

We had the good fortune to raise a beautiful black lab that we eventually named Hart. We were given a letter of the alphabet, and ours was the letter H. We selected several names for our new girl, but eventually Hart was the name the organization gave approval to. What a joy those eighteen months were, packed with so many wonderful memories. She was a great addition to our family and brought a lot of spunk as well as being a good friend for Puppy and Shrimp.

Even more important, it was a great time for Corey, who fell in love with Hart the moment he met her. It was wonderful to watch them bond and grow. He took all his responsibilities in stride and never seemed to mind when he had to wake up with her several times a night. Even at his Bar Mitzvah, she was the guest of honor. In fact, the theme of his Bar Mitzvah was the quote "B'hol l'vaveha," which is from Deuteronomy 6:4–9. B'hol l'vaveha means "With All Your Heart." On the cover of the special booklet we prepared for this momentous occasion was printed a heart. Within the heart was a special bar mitzvah photograph of Corey and Hart. Hart looked adorable. She was so cute in her skullcap, one made just for her.

Hart was always at Corey's side, and on this day it was obvious she needed to be there. At the Bar Mitzvah, Hart sat next to the family, sometimes yawning and appearing bored. However, her eyes were always focused on her pal Corey. She even tried to join him on the platform when he was saying his final prayers. When Corey addressed the congregation, he spoke lovingly of his relationship with Hart. She had started out as his "mitzvah"—good deed project. But at this juncture, Hart was truly part of his soul.

We knew when we took on Hart's puppy training that she'd eventually have to leave us. What I couldn't have imagined was just how hard it would be to give her up. It is probably one of the greatest experiences we shared as a family. We watched our youngest son take such pride in the girl he had reared, and we all shared in the love she generated throughout our household. We attempted to be stoic and avoided the fact that we'd soon be missing an integral part of our lives.

The last week was horrible. Nya, my wife, was really frustrated with me. I was the adult and was supposed to be strong for my son, helping him cope with his separation. Unfortunately, that wasn't what happened. I was devastated and couldn't pretend that the exit of this little black lab wasn't breaking my heart. In an attempt to ease our pain, we gave her a going away party where a couple of family friends came by to give her their best wishes.

I had tried to prepare for the moment. Over the course of the eighteen months, I sometimes would pen letters to Corey from Hart. My son got a kick out of it. The final note "she" wrote, though, was the hardest for me. I went to a crystal shop and had them engrave a heart-shaped jewelry box which simply stated "To Corey: My favorite human being. B'hol l'vaveha: With All My Heart—I will always love you. Your Hart." Inside the heart was this note:

My Dear Corey:

Well, the time has come for us to say good-bye. I have dreaded this day, because I know you won't see me for a while. I want to make you proud of me because you worked so hard so I could become a guide dog. I promise I will do my best!!!

You are the greatest teacher. Mostly though, you have been my best friend. I loved hanging out with you. Every day has been a new adventure. Even when I get in a jam, you never got mad. You just said, "You'll get it right next time, girl." It was great to run while you roller bladed, chased balls, and sneaked cookies when Nya wasn't watching. Most of all I loved cuddling and letting you know you were my hero.

I want you to know that even though I won't be with you, I will never forget you. You have helped me to grow up to be a big girl. I would not be who I am without you. I know I have also left you with something as well. Corey, giving to others is the best gift you can ever share. You are that giver, a sweet boy who has shaped my love.

Remember one thing. Although I may not see you, I will always be in your heart forever. Thanks for loving me.

I love you. Hart.

I had a class the day Corey and my wife took Hart to Sylmar. Perhaps it was for the best because, knowing myself, I would have made things worse. In fact, I was such a mess that day that I actually forgot all my afternoon appointments. I just went for a long hike, the hike I had always taken with Hart and Puppy. At five o'clock that afternoon I remembered the things I was supposed to have done. I scrambled, calling my patients and apologizing. They all understood—although I was a therapist, I was human too.

Over the next six weeks, I would call and see how she was doing with her training. She was doing great, and we were all proud of her. Although I missed her, I realized that in a short while she would be helping someone in need, and this gave me a sense of relief and satisfaction. This was, after all, the whole point of undertaking Hart's care.

Many of my clients also became very attached to Hart. Unlike her golden stepsister (Puppy), Hart was a lot more independent, but definitely as loving. I recall one boy, Bobby, who really enjoyed Hart's company while in therapy. Bobby had a severe form of Tourette's syndrome and was also coping with the divorce of his parents. When he found out Hart was leaving, he was upset for himself, but very concerned for my well-being. He said, "Dr. Fine, I know you will be lost without her. I can see it in your eyes. Don't lie to me!" He then told me that he would write Santa and only ask for a new black Lab for Dr. Fine.

As it turned out, Christmas that year was rich with two gifts. Two days before the holidays I got a phone call from Guide Dogs, sharing good and bad news. The bad news was that in Hart's final physical exam it was determined that she had a mild heart murmur. Ironic isn't it, that the dog that was named after the organ of life would have a mild disorder? The disorder wasn't too dangerous, but it would prevent her from being a guide dog. The good news was that we could adopt her if we wanted.

I dropped everything I was doing that afternoon and drove immediately to pick her up. It was a reunion I will never forget. You should have seen me. I ran to Hart and didn't let her go. Although Corey was her true trainer, she had a lot of me in her as well. She licked the tears of joy off my face. I smiled and told her, "You're coming home for good." A feeling of great joy came over me. I couldn't wait to get her home so we could all romp and be together again. Although she wasn't able to be a service dog, my patients would be blessed because she would become one of the "therapy girls."

A day later, into my office comes Bobby with a huge stuffed animal that looked like a black lab . He told me Santa wasn't able to find the perfect match, but he had brought this beautiful stuffed dog to help me cherish the love I had with Hart. He was smiling so much when he gave me the gift. I looked at him with a big smile of my own and said, "Thanks for making my holiday the greatest!" Then, as if on cue, Hart came running down the hallway and greeted Bobby and the huge stuffed dog. You should have seen his eyes. His Santa wish really had come true. From then on, he always called Hart "his girl" since it was because of him that Santa had brought back our "heart."

PJ

She is our second-youngest dog, and we got her six months after Puppy's death. She is as cute as a button and sweet. What can I tell you about PJ? When Puppy died, it was as if I had lost my best friend. We had been together for so many years. She had been with me nearly all day, everyday. In fact, my friends nicknamed Puppy "My Girlfriend" because she was always around. My wife always found that commentary quite amusing. "Another woman I could fight, but a dog—well. I don't have a chance."

Puppy's death caused a true emptiness. We had been together for ten years, and I felt as though I had lost a soul mate as well as a good friend. Many encouraged me to get a new dog quickly because they felt it would help me cope with the loss. I strongly disagreed and felt it would be a long time before I would ever want another animal of any kind. But my family, especially my boys, were committed to changing my mind. After several months, and without my knowledge, they made

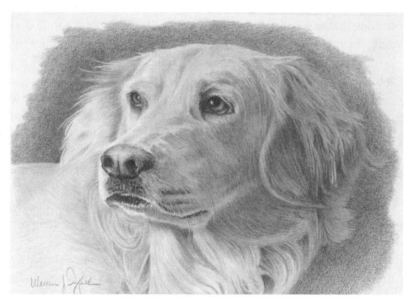

contact with several breeders to find me a new puppy. Everyone in the family was in on it.

On the first night of Hanukah that year, the boys presented me with a card. It said, "Happy Hanukah, Dad. We don't have your gift in the envelope, but this is the best present we will ever give you. We will get to see your 'golden' smile again because this is a certificate for a new 'Golden Puppy' who isn't yet born." They watched me for a few moments to assess my reaction. I was speechless at first, and then tears dripped from the corners of my eyes.

They knew better than I what was needed, and that very evening I called the breeder to discuss the birth of my new puppy. Over the next few months I visited the mom weekly and got to know her temperament. Sundance was a beautiful show dog. She also had degrees in obedience and tracking. Her coloring was absolutely beautiful; she was a light golden color and had terrific people skills. My heart beat a little faster just being in contact with this golden retriever and anticipating the birth of my new dog.

Three months later I witnessed the birth of her litter, falling immediately in love with a light blond golden that was identified only with a red piece of yarn around her neck. Over the course of the next eight weeks, I would visit "Ms. Red" and play with her and her siblings. She also had a wonderful temperament; she wasn't passive, but on the other hand, she wasn't as domineering as her siblings. My weekly visits strengthened my love for Ms. Red. The more I got to know her, the more excited I was to take her home.

To share my excitement, I began posting pictures of Ms. Red at my office. My patients also were excited about the new puppy and were eagerly awaiting her arrival. To engage their involvement, I solicited name suggestions for Ms. Red. Over a few weeks many suggestions were given such as Hope, Blondie, and Jubilee. One of my eleven-year-old patients made a touching suggestion. He wrote: "I have the best name in the world, Dr. Fine. Why not name her PJ? Although she will grow up and be her own dog, naming her Puppy Jr. (alias PJ) will allow her to keep Puppy's spirit alive." On that day, Ms. Red became PJ. I thought this was perfect, that we'd come full circle.

PJ didn't come to the office for any extended period of time until she was several months old. However, once she had all her shots, I thought it would be okay for her to make quick visits. Before PJ's arrival on that morning, I prepared the office for almost two hours. I also spruced up the porch so that when she went outside it would be sparkling clean. Her favorite chew toys were scattered all over the two back rooms. On April 14 we drove to the office at about 3 p.m. Hart escorted PJ into the office and was there to show her the ropes. I'm not sure how much she helped, but it was cute to watch the senior mentor the rookie.

Magic

When our good friends asked us the question: "Do you want to have one of our puppies when they arrive?" The answer was a definite "No." Nya especially felt that three dogs were enough. But as the month approached for the puppies to be born, our friends asked one more time: "Don't you want one of Maples' puppies?" Nya thought about it and replied, "Our oldest dog, Shrimp, is fourteen years old, Hart is ten, and PJ is six. No, I do not need any more dogs, the answer remains the same."

Nya goes on to explain:

A few weeks later and for some unknown reason, I started actually thinking about it. When I spoke to Aubrey, he could not believe it. I think he was beginning to worry about me for even thinking about it. He knows how adamant I have been whenever the subject comes up. When I made my decision, everyone was shocked, including me. All the negative reasons definitely outweighed the positive ones, but the family was going to get a new pup. We decided to name her Magic.

When the puppies were born, we were discussing which one was cute, which one was mellow, which one was too excitable. In the end, I think we made a great choice. As we waited for the pups to mature, my family and friends were still in a state of shock. If I heard it once, I heard it a hundred times—"I can't believe you said yes." I could not explain it to myself. Something just told me to go ahead and get the new pup.

When it was time to bring Magic home, Aubrey was out of town, so I was busy preparing things. Everyone knows how much you have to get ready for a new pup, and you better not be short of energy. I was ready for the cute little Magic, but a tough job was ahead of me. I remember when the other dogs were pups, and I thought, "Why am I doing this?"

During this week of preparation, I went for an ultra-sound as a follow-up to my yearly mammogram. They explained that they wanted to do a biopsy. They had an opening that

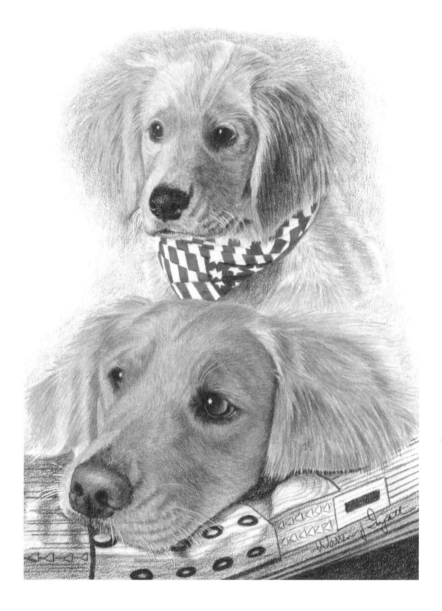

afternoon, and I wanted to get it done as soon as possible, knowing that after Magic's arrival time would be crunched. This occurred on Tuesday, and by Friday I was diagnosed with breast cancer. All of a sudden I knew why I was getting this puppy.

I decided not to tell anyone until after I met with the sur-

geon. I wanted to know exactly what the scenario would be so I could answer questions when my family and friends asked. As I drove to pick up Magic, I was filled with anxiety. Not knowing what was going to happen to me or how to tell my family and friends was beginning to overwhelm me. I knew I could cover up my feelings when I was around people, but I was scared.

When I arrived, Magic was full of pep and roaming around the house like she owned it. I knew my work was cut out for me. She ran up to me, gave a quick sniff, and was off again running. Finally in her crate, it was time for the long drive home. As I backed out, Magic began to whimper. I told her I knew how she felt. I was scared too. Our relationship began at this moment. Two scared souls looking for comfort from one another. I found a best friend who was going to help me through this event in my life. The journey was just beginning.

Celebrations

Everyday life with a pack of dogs, not to mention the birds, fish, and lizards, is always interesting. Life outside of my office is quite different and, frankly, frequently a challenge as well as a joy. Part of my family's foundation is that we love to party, to celebrate even the smallest event or accomplishment, and this includes our animals. To help celebrate PJ's first birthday, we threw a large party for her. In attendance were about fifty children. It was amazing. What surprised me was how excited they were to come. Each of them brought PJ a birthday present. When I asked one girl why she brought her a present, she looked at me and said, "How can you come to a birthday party without a present?"

The afternoon was filled with lots of activities and PJ just wandered around greeting her guests. On one side of the parking lot we set up a food area; we called it PJ's Café, and a few of the parents helped grill hot dogs and hamburgers. When PJ was presented with her large birthday cookie, she didn't know what to do at first. When she finally realized that it was for her, she gobbled her treat, and after only seconds, her muzzle was covered in icing.

For her next birthday we decided to let Hart share center stage, since her birthday is only two weeks after PJ's. The special event was celebrated by inviting approximately twenty-five of the dogs' girlfriends for a British tea party. I have to confess that I really enjoyed setting that one up. For a couple of weeks I went shopping and bought cheap china so that every child seated had her own china place setting.

I had a few of my college students help me organize the party, and they were as excited as I was. They had never been to a party where the guests of honor had four paws.

But they had experience with hosting parties for little girls, and they recommended the activities and the atmosphere. We had three stations that the girls could visit. One station was the crafts area, where guests could make birthday cards for PJ and Hart or make decoupage candles.

The parents and children helped with the food preparation and their contributions were fantastic—small heart-shaped egg sandwiches and bone-shaped ones filled with peanut butter. In addition, we also had chocolate covered strawberries, cookies, and, of course, tea and hot chocolate. The girls took attending PJ and Hart's celebration very seriously, wearing their best "tea" dresses.

Of course the guests of honor were also amazed with the food and activity at the party. When the guests arrived, we had a photo booth set up where the girls could take pictures with the dogs. To make the pictures more amusing, we had the dogs put brightly colored boas on. For entertainment, I put on a magic show for all the guests.

To many it may seem odd to shower lavish attention on our animals, but I believe the celebrations for our animal family members are a great way to show children and adults the power of positive actions. So I continue the tradition. When Magic turned one year old, we decided to have a party for her and her littermates. We had little trouble convincing our friend, and the owner of Magic's mother, to go along with it. She, along with one of her friends, decided to host the party so that all the littermates could attend. Each family brought treats for dogs and humans alike. We still can't believe the experience of that party. The dogs played together as if they had never been apart. The adults shared a year's worth of stories, and we even managed to get a large "family" photo taken. It was wonderful to watch Magic play with her brothers and sisters, and this brought home to everyone who attended just how important family really is. I even heard many of the adults talk about arranging their own family reunions.

The Antics: Home Isn't Always Shangri-la

Although the dogs are pretty obedient and well-trained for office work, they often get themselves into jams or mischief at home. This can range from sneaking out of the house to, at times, even swiping food. I will never forget late one night when I heard lots of barking outside. The barking was coming from down the street, and I remember rolling over and telling Nya how irresponsible the owners were to allow their dogs to make such racket. I said this with an owner's confidence in knowing that his dogs were tucked away safely. I was wrong. We had just re-carpeted the entire house, and, because of the mess we had left the dogs on the back porch. Since I was awake, I decided to check on our dogs and to my surprise, I found the back gate was wide open and all the dogs (Goldie, Puppy, Shrimp and Hart) were gone. Once I realized it was my dogs causing the ruckus, I immediately raced out of the house in only my boxer shorts and t-shirt. There they were, howling at all the other dogs fenced in their yards. Shrimp and Goldie looked like they were having the best time. They were strutting their stuff like two big shots. All of them looked startled when I caught them in their naughty act. I could see they didn't want to stop, but like a chain gang they followed each other back into the house. Once at home, I decided to corral them in our bedroom. "What is that smell?" Nya asked immediately. I was caught off guard because I didn't smell anything. As the dogs lingered in the room, the potency of the smell grew stronger. Nya got out of bed and said, "It's Shrimp. Can't you smell him? He's been sprayed by a skunk." Getting closer to him, I could smell his distinct aroma. I immediately took him outside. The next morning we cleaned him up and he smelled as good as new, but it would be a night none of us would forget.

Sneaking food is also a behavior that all the dogs have been guilty of. My favorite recollection stems from one of my clients, Derek, and my birthday celebration. On my birthday Derek and his mother brought me a pizza with the works. It smelled wonderful! When they arrived we spoke for a few moments, but I had to get ready for my next appointment. I thanked the family and I told Derek to put the pizza on the table in the back.

Puppy was with me that day, but her help wasn't needed the whole time and she wandered in and out. After a few hours, I told a client about the pizza and offered him a piece. When we walked into the back room, I found what had occupied Puppy's free time. She was on the floor, her legs crossed in front of her holding one of the last pieces of pizza. She looked at me with innocent eyes. I chuckled for a while, but was a little upset that I missed out on my treat. That night Puppy drank bowl after bowl of water, which meant trip after trip outside. So, I also paid the price for her gluttony but without having had the pleasure.

Then there's Hart, who on occasion also has transgressed. One memorable time occurred when she came back from Guide Dog Training. Nya was finishing barbecuing a meal and left two cooked steaks on the kitchen counter. When Nya returned to the kitchen, the steaks were nowhere to be found. After a little detective work, she found Hart eating the last morsel. I must admit Nya was not as amused with this incident as I was with Puppy's pizza escapade.

In fact, sneaking food, for some unknown reason, happens more in Nya's presence than mine. On another occasion, Nya had been eating a tostada but was called away from the table. When she returned to her plate, she found PJ sitting in her chair and eating her meal. When PJ noticed that Nya had come back, she jumped off the chair, tostada filling her mouth, and began to run. The pursuit must have been hysterical, PJ leading Nya on a merry chase as she pleaded with PJ to relinquish her prize.

I was so amused by the incident that during an afternoon session later that day I told one of my clients about it. Mitchell couldn't stop laughing. In fact, even to this day he brings up the PJ story and has a good laugh. Although many of these events are amusing and some are exasperating, they are lessons. I've learned patience, the importance of disciplining with love, and that failures also teach us about ourselves. Believe me when I say that my dogs are angels, but often they get their wings clipped. Life on my ranch is both bitter and sweet, but this is to be expected, this is life. We look for sunshine every morning, but occasionally we encounter rain. Do we put on a raincoat and grab our umbrella and venture forth or stay home? I advocate going out. Getting wet is not so bad; after all, the sun always returns to dry us off.

PJ's Bark Insight

Magic and I went to Fallbrook last winter for a week's visit with our second family. Our two-leggers went on a trip to Mexico. Life at the Berl's can be a dog's dream come true. We get the royal golden treatment. Snacks, walks and even a snooze in the big bed are some of the perks. Lance and Stephanie are the two people who convinced Aubrey many years ago that goldens were great family dogs. We are thankful to them because without their input we may have never joined the family. Magic's mom, Maple, lives there, so whenever Magic goes down to Fallbrook it is like old home week for all of us.

In Fallbrook, we can almost get away with anything. We get spoiled rotten. From morning to evening we hear how great we are. All day long we heard: "Where are my cute puppy dogs?" Stephanie made sure we had lots of goodies and toys. After a few days, Momma Maple tires of the kid, especially when the kid tries to grab her favorite toys. Stephanie often comes to Magic's rescue and tells Maple "share with your cute daughter, she'll only be here for a few more days."

I love the space at their house. They have lots of land so there is lots of space for running, digging and discovery. They live right next to an avocado grove, which is like paradise. While romping we get the chance to munch on some of the avocados which have fallen from the trees. They are delicious. Thank goodness I don't live here permanently. Otherwise my girlish figure would be gone.

Well into the week I noticed that Magic wasn't herself. I could tell that she was getting homesick because she wasn't as playful and skipped a few meals. Stephanie thought she was sick and sat with her to try and encourage her to eat. I should have told her not to worry. Magic wasn't physically ill, but her young heart was feeling confused. Although she was having fun, she missed our two-leggers. All she wanted to do was go home and see the gang.

Once Nya came by to get us, Magic's personality changed instantaneously. She was jumping for joy and ready to leave. She grabbed her leash and ran towards the car. She stuck next to Nya like glue that day. I thought she would get over it quickly, but I was wrong. Once we got home she still wasn't that playful. All she wanted to do is stay in our room and lay on her bed. It was almost as if she was saying, "I don't want to leave here ever again." Magic missed everyone. She didn't just miss the two-leggers, but Hart and Shrimp as well.

Although young, Magic can teach all of us a lesson: Appreciate what you have while you have it. Be happy with your loved ones and cherish them like your most valuable jewels. Family is crucial and we need to work on getting along. I believe that is what Magic was trying to tell us. There is no place like home, especially your own! Dorothy learned this in Oz, and Aubrey learned it while in Kenya. I know I wouldn't trade my life for anyone's out there. Let the partying continue! And for those of you who think a dog's life is hard, I'll let you be the judge.

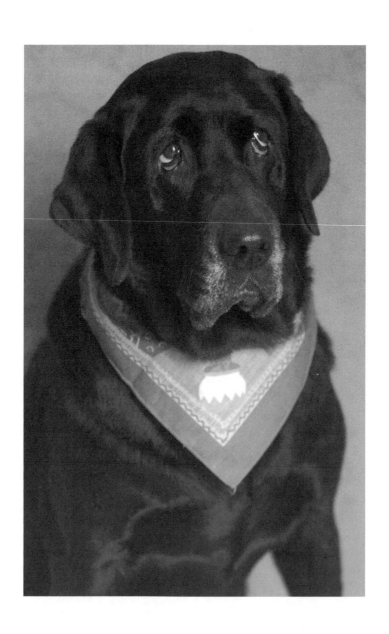

Giving from the Hart

Becoming a Comforter and a Human Builder

On Sarah's first office visit after her release from the hospital, she is more at ease but still reserved. As we sit and talk, Hart sits close to her chair. At one point in our session, Sarah's reserve finally crumbles. Pushing up her left sleeve, she shows me her scars. As she lowers her arm, Sarah notices that Hart's eyes are fixed on that arm. At that moment, Hart lifts her gaze from Sarah's arm and connects with her eyes. Hart then looks over at me with an expression on her face that I can only call puzzled, Hart looks back at Sarah, and then Hart lowers her head and begins to lick the scars. Sarah is startled for a moment but then sits quietly as Hart continues to lick the wounds. Finally, she bends over Hart and holds her close.

Although no words are spoken, I can tell that something has changed in Sarah. It is as if she has said, "I am sorry I did this, and now that we all know, we can talk about it, and I can learn to never do this again." This moment with Hart is a catalyst for a major breakthrough.

From that point on, our progress accelerated. Sarah and I talked about why she cut herself and she was honest about it for the first time. Over the next eight months, Sarah made numerous changes in her life. She began a home-school program that reduced the anxiety she had felt in a large-school setting. Once she felt more at ease, her academic performance improved dramatically. She began to volunteer at a nursery school, and this activity was helpful in dissolving her self-imposed shell. The preschool was located in a local YWCA, and sometimes she stayed there and interacted with other teens.

Along with volunteering at the YWCA, Sarah spent time helping at the local animal shelter. She explained that it made her sad to see the animals' conditions and the circumstances that brought them to the shelter. But Sarah also saw how happy they were when she gave them attention. We discussed her animal shelter experiences in our sessions together—in particular how it feels to be abandoned and how important it is to give the animals a second chance in life. She especially related to the latter because she believed she was getting a second chance too. Even more importantly, the act of helping others convinced her that she had value as a person.

For Sarah, animals were the key to her transformation. Her connection with Hart grew stronger and stronger as the weeks went by. When she visited, she made a special effort to give Hart a lot of attention. She seemed to enjoy teasing me, saying that although PJ (at the time a puppy) was cute and popular with most of the children, Hart was the greatest because she was calm, loyal and, steady.

Becoming a Comforter

Spontaneity makes actions more sincere and realistic, including actions taken by animals. But their independent actions spark questions. Why did Hart lick Sarah's wounds? Hart certainly couldn't know why Sarah had cut herself or what these cuts symbolized to her. And yet, this action brought about a turning point for Sarah.

Sarah was thirteen when we first meet. She entered with a baseball cap pulled low on her head and used the brim of the cap to cover her eyes. I saw that she was overweight, and was trembling with anxiety and fright. When I greeted her, her voice was just above a whisper. Sarah, like most of the children I work with, felt isolated and unlovable.

When Sarah and I started her therapy, I knew only what I'd learned from my initial interview with Sarah's mother. She'd told me of Sarah's problems with her family: her parents had recently divorced and her mom had taken a job outside the home, which left Sarah and her sister alone much of the time. Also she was fighting with her younger sister, and she rarely saw her older brother. This meant Sarah lacked a significant male figure in her life. In addition, Sarah's hormones and body were changing, affecting her moods and adding to her depression.

Although talking therapy has its benefits, there is something about the animals working by my side that reaches through my patients' self-imposed walls and allows them to give and receive love and care. Unlike Puppy and PJ, who sometimes seeks attention, Hart never asks. She doesn't nudge a leg or lick a hand. Therefore, on Sarah's first visit Hart simply went to her side, ready to be petted if and when Sarah felt like it. Sarah didn't look at Hart or mention the dog's presence, but after a few seconds, she did reach out and stroked Hart's head. She petted the dog without much show of emotion, and I saw that she primarily used the action of petting Hart to avoid looking at me. Yet her trembling decreased. The physical contact with Hart eased her tension and anxiety.

Sarah and I spent the first three sessions getting acquainted. We'd start our visits in the waiting room—Sarah sitting huddled in one of the chairs, the brim of her cap over her eyes. She'd continue to speak quietly and at times trembled with fear. The only time she relaxed was when she touched Hart. This was a mixed blessing, as I realize that it not only gave her comfort, but also gave her an excuse to ignore me.

Although I train my therapy dogs to respond to voice commands and hand signals, they often initiate contact and respond independently. I have found this self-initiation to be beneficial, and I have learned how to effectively manage both the animals' and the clients' behavior. A therapist working with animals in a psychological practice must know how to handle situations like Sarah's. On some occasions a patient uses an animal as a shield, hiding behind the interaction with the animal in an attempt to refocus the therapy. This is done as a means of avoidance. As I became more experienced with working alongside the animals, I began to recognize this potential pitfall.

At times, and as a temporary measure because the person feels too much stress, a detour can be healthy. However, if I ever feel that a patient's interaction with an animal sidetracks the real focus of therapy, I intervene. Over the years, the dogs have become aware of my reactions to their behavior in the office. They frequently "check in" with me during our sessions. When I believe that their presence has become too much of a distraction, I signal for them to stop engaging and they just step back from the situation.

In Sarah's case, she used Hart initially as a shield because we were just getting to know each other. Hart acted as a social lubricant, easing Sarah's anxiety and fear. During our early sessions she petted Hart and listened to me, but divulged little. It felt as if we were treading water, but I didn't want to push her. My goal was to build a relationship with this seriously withdrawn girl—a relationship that she trusted. Allowing Sarah to choose this course of action slowed our progress, but in the end, it was a more effective tool. Although our progress was slow, I did learn more about Sarah during the early sessions.

At one session she stated, "I have no real friends and feel like an outcast. They ignore me because I'm different. They can't see my fear, that I'm just afraid all the time." Adding to her fear was the high incidence of violence and crime in her neighborhood. Because of this, she felt her two primary environments, home and school, held no comfort or safety. To help deal with her fear, she wore clothes that she could hide in: an oversized army jacket, matching army green pants, sneakers, and always a baseball cap pulled low over her eyes. To make matters worse, Sarah wasn't sleeping well; she stayed up all night, sitting at her computer or watching television. In addition to reinforcing her isolation, her lack of sleep was undermining her mental and physical health.

Things with Sarah came to a head after our third session. Since she hadn't made measurable progress and was still demoralized, she retreated farther and farther inside herself. Then Sarah began to cut herself on the arm, initially using a pin but soon moved to using a razor. She kept her wounds hidden from everyone, but eventually showed her arm to another girl at school, who became frightened and told the counselor. For Sarah's safety, the counselor immediately placed Sarah in a psychiatric facility. Sarah was devastated and frightened. But it also was the turning point in our relationship.

Once in the hospital and surrounded by other competent and sympathetic mental health providers, she told them she wanted to call me. When Sarah and I talked, I told her that this experience could be good for her—at least for a short while. She needed to work through her challenges, and I encouraged her to work with the doctors but to call if she needed me. Over the course of the next couple of weeks she called regularly to let me know how she was doing. Although this hospitalization was a setback, I was pleased. Hart and I had won her trust.

After Sarah's release from the facility, our sessions resumed, along with walking the dogs, Hart and PJ, which became an important part of our afternoons together. Sarah loved having the chance to walk Hart, and her special affection for the dog helped initiate a new openness in our discussions. We chatted together while the dogs trotted ahead of us. On these walks, I often perched my umbrella cockatoo, Snowflake, on my shoulder, and Sarah got a real kick out of this.

It was amusing to watch Snowflake sidle in for the walks. She was as excited as the dogs. Once she witnessed the gang getting on their leashes, she'd hop onto the cage's door, a cue to let me know she was ready and willing. Once the walk began, she bobbed her head in excitement and vocalized, to the delight of the youngsters.

Our walk led us to a park near my office, and here I saw an entirely new side to Sarah. She giggled while she played with Hart—rubbing the dog's belly and scratching her head. Sometimes the two dogs romped together, and Sarah enjoyed watching the two dogs playfully engage. When Hart got excited, not only did she wag her tail, but her back end also began to wag, going from side to side in a comical doggy rumba. This sight always made Sarah laugh. I noticed, though, that at the same time Hart stayed attuned to Sarah and gave her full attention by frequently pausing to check on her. During these walks, the trembling, fear, and anxiety Sarah exhibited in my office disappeared. She became more at ease, which was the primary reason for our walks. The casual atmosphere made her feel less confined and stressed.

While we were able to discuss her progress while walking the dogs, the office remained our primary therapy setting. At difficult moments during our office sessions, Sarah would hold on to Hart. It was only then—with the help of a security blanket in the shape of a black Labrador—that she'd speak out about what she needed. Over the course of the next eight months, Sarah's progress was amazing. She was more open to talking about her life, and the shell that surrounded her began to crumble.

Sarah had been placed in a special school program, and her progress in this modified system was tremendous and her thirst for knowledge had been invigorated. She ventured out of her circle of comfort and socialized with peers. This area was the slowest to develop, but everyone saw improvement. Slowly, we began to see less of each other, until one afternoon we agreed she could be on her own.

It had been over two years since I had heard from or seen Sarah, when one day, out of the blue, I received a wonderful email from her. She wrote:

Hello Dr. Fine:

You may not remember me, but I was "seeing" you for a while when I was younger. I was doing research about animals in psychology and I read about a book you were writing about your animals. It reminded me of how when I had "seen" you, I was so scared and nervous about saying the wrong thing, that I usually didn't talk about much. I remember how whenever I was nervous, Hart and Shrimp would be right there, as if telling me that you're not a "bad" guy and the such. Hart especially seemed to be the one being the psychologist, always sitting near me, comforting me from everything that I would worry about. She is what I remember most about my visits.

49

She also gave me an excuse to talk to my Mom about what was going on at the time.

In the end, I don't remember talking to you about much, but all that I did tell you was for those two . . . and some of the fish (though one isn't able to pet a fish) and the bearded dragon. My Mom and I still talk about one of the fish in the waiting room that would swim in a repetitive motion, and looked like it was the happiest fish in the world, and I still tell my friends about how I went on a walk with a bird. (They still don't believe me.)

I hope all is well with you and the animals. Good luck on the book.

I was in Holland when I read her email, sitting in a small Internet café. My eyes welled up as I reflected about our times together. Her letter moved me. Perhaps the most significant reason was that she let me know how she was doing and acknowledged our efforts in her transformation. I don't help people for the thank-you they give, but when I do get it, I am touched. The email solidified my beliefs about why Sarah and I had connected. The animals and I, together with the help of her family, the school, and the volunteer agencies, helped to build a support system for Sarah that allowed her to flourish and grow. More specifically, it was Hart's ability to establish a comfort zone for Sarah that eventually got her to open up and give life a chance.

Six months after her email, I invited Sarah to my office to chat and get reacquainted.

She looks quite different. Her hair is longer, she is wearing glasses, and there is a positive air in the way she carries herself. She looks confident. She sits more comfortably in the chair, and there is a simple but beautiful glow in her eyes. She now speaks clearly and her voice is strong.

Hart wanders over to Sarah, just the way she used to. Her tail is wagging and her body sways back and forth. Sarah looks into Hart's eyes and says, "You are the one who got me through the tough time. You got me to talk." It is a touching moment. They embrace, as though no time has passed and Hart is still the blanket of fur that comforts her. It is evident that Hart remembers her.

Sarah was excited to tell me all about her accomplishments. But even more she delighted in telling me about her new life. She was a full-time student at a local high school, earning A's and B's. Additionally, since going back to school she had become more outgoing, joining a hiking club and an animal advocacy and support group. She told me she has become a member of a service group that raises money to send livestock to underdeveloped countries. For a short while she explained her love of all these new opportunities, but then she focused more on her relationships with people. "I like the volunteer work with the animals, but I like hanging out with friends more. I've met a girl with some of my problems and I try to help her because I know the pitfalls."

For Sarah, being more outgoing and joining groups was new, and her excitement was comparable to a child entering a candy store for the first time. She was in awe of all her new options. At one point in the afternoon, Sarah was more reflective and spoke of her past life and how she felt separated from others and empty inside. "It was like a glass divided the world into two. I was on the other side and couldn't get in." She then took her eyes off of me and stared deeply at Hart. She said, "Hart and you helped me get on the path that opened the world up for me. It is funny that it was a dog that taught me to talk." A few minutes later she left. Although I haven't heard from her since, the images of a more secure and happy young woman has stayed with me.

Therapy animals can act as a buffer for clients, making it easier for them to cope, and Sarah's experience is not uncommon. One memorable event took place a couple of years ago, with a girl named Gail.

————

It is about 4:00 p.m. on a Friday afternoon. Gail arrives for her weekly visit bursting with anger. For years she has been the brunt of everyone's jokes and feels like an outcast in a school. Today, she is angry at the world and enters the office ranting at her parents and me. "I want to go home! I told you I didn't want to come today. I'm tired and fed up with everybody! What can you do anyways? You can't stop them from bugging me! They aren't fair. Everyone blames me for any problems. They always just start up with me."

It takes a while until I can convince her to walk back to one of the therapy rooms. Once we leave the waiting room, Gail's anger continues to fester. I try to begin a conversation, but Gail avoids our discussion by covering her face with her hands. Although I sense her irritation and frustration, I wonder if she is trying to provoke a confrontation deliberately. Is she hoping to alienate me, and thus build more walls? Being unpopular and being aware of it is hard for her or any child to cope with. She sits with her head down, hopeless of any resolution. She doesn't want to talk, and only the sound of sobbing can be heard throughout my office.

I am not sure how to proceed. I want to be helpful, and if she would let me, I know we could work together. However, her response thus far makes me feel less optimistic. After a few moments of sobbing, PJ engages Gail by resting her head in the girl's lap. Gail resists PJ's affection, and so she trots over to her bed. But PJ's big brown eyes are tranquilizing and inviting, even from across the room.

Gail walks over to PJ's bed and curls up next to her. I'm surprised, and I realize that today is going to be different. Gail is like a child holding on to a beloved teddy bear, and PJ seems to sense Gail's pain and lies still as she is being held. Her brown eyes gaze into Gail's and for the next few moments they communicate in silence. Not a word is said between them, but in their silence comfort is found. I allow this contact to continue for several minutes. I then sit down on the carpet nearby.

I spoke to her of loneliness and feeling left out. After a few minutes of hearing only my voice, I heard a soft whisper. She never left PJ's side, but with PJ's help I was able to help Gail verbalize some of her feelings of demoralization and loneliness. "Why me, why me?" she said over and over. "Even when I try, they never give me a chance. The teachers never believe me when I complain. They always take the other kids' side." I listened without commenting, allowing Gail the opportunity to vent now that she was less agitated and had acknowledged my presence as a sounding board rather than an antagonist.

The session proved more productive than I anticipated, but we still had much more to resolve. Eventually, Gail got over her self-pity and was open to discussing ways to make a difference.

Gail and PJ became close therapy buddies over the next few months. During our visits, she continued to seek out PJ's company, and PJ reciprocated with love and loyalty as she remained by Gail's side for every visit. Over the months, Gail began to appreciate her own assets and started to find joy in life. As she made substantial progress, our visits become fewer.

When I first began working with animals, I was impressed initially with their innate talent in establishing warm and strong relationships with the clients. My appreciation for their natural gifts was enlightened even further when I began to grasp how much more they could contribute. They were not merely living "teddy bears" but purposeful creatures that acted with tremendous sensitivity and kindness. These co-therapists are intuitive about the needs of humans, even though they communicate differently. Their actions come from their hearts and souls. I sit in awe as I witness how the animals gauge a client's mood. When they notice clients in despair, their knack of comforting comes to the forefront.

Animals as comforters come in all shapes and reassure in different ways. A colleague who lives in Orange County has a seven-year-old female golden retriever that he uses as a therapy dog in a school for educating children with emotional difficulties. Teddy is a true sweetheart, and over the years she has become one of PJ's best buddies. Teddy is somewhat dark for a golden retriever and her most distinctive feature are the blonde "feathers" on her legs and chest. She began working at the school when she was three years old. The staff sees her as a relaxing and calming influence for the children, and they love having Teddy as a member of their classes.

But this isn't an example of how Teddy comforted the students. It is much more. One day a meeting was called to review and plan for the emotional needs of one particular student who was having great difficulty at the school. The boy had been abused and traumatized in his early years and was removed from his biological family. He was adopted, but the family members were overwhelmed and sometimes misunderstood their son's behaviors. Over the years, with only minimal gains, both the parents and the staff were becoming discouraged.

At this meeting over fifteen professionals gathered to discuss their perceptions of why this boy was having numerous problems. The boy was not present at the meeting, but his adoptive father was there. Also at the meeting was Teddy, asleep on the floor.

———

For over an hour the father sits silently, overwhelmed with all the information and opinions he is hearing. He feels alone, as if stranded in the eye of a hurricane. Adding to the family's stress is the father's recent recovery from a stroke, and this meeting finds him still adjusting to his disability. When he speaks his voice is weak. Unfortunately for him, the others in the room are oblivious to his condition, confusion, and fears as they continue with the discussion and commentary. It is only Teddy who is conscious of the father's uneasiness. She gets up from her corner and sits next to him and begins licking his hand. She looks up and gazes at the rest of the people in the room. Is she trying to scold them and make them aware of this man's doubts and discomfort?

Staff members in the room are embarrassed at Teddy's actions and feel it negates the professional nature of the meeting. A staff member gives a command for Teddy to stop and return to the corner. At the father's insistence, though, Teddy is allowed to stay by his side for the rest of the meeting. The father states he needs her reassurance and support. It is Teddy that is giving the man empathy, comfort, and encouragement to continue listening and speaking about his adopted son. It is Teddy that acts as his safe zone, and she helps him through this difficult time.

What had Teddy seen or sensed that the humans had missed? Why did she feel it was necessary to get up and and console the father while the others sat back and didn't respond to his needs? These, after all, were trained mental health providers, and they should have been sensitive to this man's needs. Had they grown callous over the years and become immune to these feelings? Unfortunately, some professionals feel flustered when emotions are evoked and don't react appropriately. All they needed to do was acknowledge his pain and allow him to grieve, both for his son and himself. What harm would there have been to act more humanely and provide this man, this father, with a little tender support and understanding?

I can appreciate this story. When I began my career, I easily could have made the same mistake. Sometimes, as a therapist, I found myself focusing so intently on what needs to be said that I directed the conversation and focus in too tightly on the facts, unfortunately jeopardizing the emotions. However, I learned early that to do my job well, I needed to be flexible and not follow a script. Rather, I needed to demonstrate that compassion and care are primary to not only the patient, but also the family. If this means a meeting takes longer, so be it.

This is so important that I now find myself explaining difficult and challenging issues to families while in the company of the dogs. As I do so, the dogs sit vigilantly, ready to give comfort if needed. They make these encounters less sterile and more attuned to individual needs. But this lesson of giving comfort and affording safety can be applied outside of the professional setting. When I allowed myself this flexibility, it also became clear to me that my life outside of my office could also benefit, especially as a parent. We owe it to ourselves to become more humane and sensitive to others in all areas of life.

Learning to be open and sensitive to the needs of others doesn't have to be limited to professionals working in mental health. Just as each of us must have a sense of comfort and safety in our daily lives, we also have the capacity to learn to be more open and sensitive to those around us. We may not have loved ones experiencing situations similar to Sarah, Gail, and the father mentioned in this chapter, but certainly there are days when we either feel especially in need of comfort or know of someone who is. The needs may range from having a bad day at work or a misunderstanding between friends, to more prolonged trouble, such as a death or divorce.

If you know of someone who is depressed, lonely, or experiencing a difficult challenge, take a minute and ask yourself how you might help. Sending a cheerful card, stopping by for a short visit, or phoning for a quick chat won't take much of your time but could be just the tonic someone else needs. You might also consider sharing your pet with a friend in need by taking your animal along for a short visit. If you're a parent or grandparent of a child like Sarah, consider buying a pet. The wonderful thing about pets is that even though they come in all shapes, kinds, and sizes and with varying degrees of care required, they all have the potential for sharing love and comfort. For the best results, you'll want to choose wisely, taking into account the requirements of different species and breeds as well as your family members' temperaments and schedules.

Becoming a Human Builder

One of the reasons why I wanted to become a therapist was that I enjoy helping others. When I was a teenager, if anyone had asked me what I wanted to be when I grew up, I would have said, even then, that I wanted to work with children, perhaps even become a psychologist. What I couldn't have fathomed at that juncture was that my life would cross paths with a group of animals that would help me do my job better. Nor did I realize that they would not only help me with my job, but also my life.

The most rewarding aspect of being a therapist is the opportunity to help others rebuild their lives. Many have been devastated because of domestic hardships, while others have become victims to life's misfortunes. The bottom line is this: therapists help build or rebuild humans. Some people call therapists shrinks. I believe this is an inaccurate term that implies intrusion and reduction. I prefer the metaphor of a human builder. Being a human builder is a much kinder and perhaps a more accurate phrase because it opens up the possibility that each of us has this potential.

The building or remodeling of a person is quite different from the development or renovation of a home. It's not as easy or simple as buying tools, wood, and cement. A human's reconstruction can't be completed or repaired with a hammer and nails. Rather, individuals require the channeling of human character, emotions, and integrity; therefore, making a difference in a person's life can be quite a challenge. Yet there is a similarity. Picture yourself standing next to a professional builder and in front of a wall that needs repair. Although you realize the work must be done, you need assurance that this professional knows what he or she is doing, especially with the first swing of that hammer.

This scenario is not unlike the first visit with a therapist. There are several unique qualities that a therapist needs to consider while helping a person remodel or rebuild. The possibilities are endless, depending on the individual and his/her personality and needs. Traits such as honesty, trustworthiness, integrity, respect for others and oneself, and forgiveness are a few important character qualities that readily come to mind. For example, helping people discover that putting down those axes they grind frees them to embrace forgiveness, a quality that will help them better contend with life. Those that can forgive find their lives easier to manage because they release themselves from the chains of the past. The same might be said, to some extent, of animals.

My own animals, some of whom have histories of neglect or abuse, have overcome their past lives by learning to trust again and, perhaps, to forgive. I frequently discuss Puppy's past with the children. She serves as an example and helps clients recognize their ability to forgive and trust once again. Like Puppy, this knowledge allows the children to move on and live a more fulfilled and loving life. A few of my birds and my bearded dragon also have similar histories. Spikey, the dragon, had part of his tail cut off, but that didn't mean she couldn't overcome it. Nevertheless, having a shorter tail is always a source for discussion. "How could anyone do that to her?" is a comment I hear from children. More often that leads into a discussion of overcoming past tragedies and in some cases dealing with or forgiving the abuser.

Other important building blocks I focus on are helping others develop a sense of humor, a sense of fairness, compassion, and kindness. If we stop to think about it, people we enjoy being around have these positive qualities. Visualize coming home from a long day and being greeted by your dog. Dogs aren't afraid to run up and let us know how important we are to them. Humans can learn a lot from these actions. Letting someone know how much you care is a tremendous gift that is best shown and appreciated through actions, however small.

Finally, the belief that "I am responsible for my day" is a message that we all can live by and is one of the foundation stones for building a healthy self-esteem. In the end, the greatest gift to my clients is helping them understand and gain insight into their own ambitions and drive. When people become too dependent on others to have their desires met, they lose out. While they need to know that we believe in them and recognize that they can get their jobs in life done, they ultimately are in charge of making things happen. Taking responsibility for ourselves is empowering and a worthwhile skill to learn.

Helping others build or shore up their sense of self can be a reciprocal process. Numerous professionals have studied what it takes to be a human builder or helper. We all learn from others. My best teachers in life haven't been the professors I studied with in ivory towers. My best teachers have been those "everyday" folks I've met and some of the animals that have surrounded me. But having a positive impact on a person's life is dependent on how the relationship is established and how it flourishes.

My most influential mentor taught me that what should matter in life isn't who you worked to be, but rather how you lived your life. When I was just a kid, my grandfather, God rest his soul, was probably the most significant influence. A tailor by trade, he was not formally educated, and because he was blind, some people underestimated his abilities and his wisdom. For most of my childhood I turned to him as my advisor. His simple approach to living demonstrated to me that my life could be rich if I believed in others and was kindhearted. These are two principles that I have taken with me, both personally and professionally.

As a young boy, I used to take short excursions with my grandfather throughout Montreal. We talked about many things, but most of all we talked about growing up and how to be a "somebody." "A somebody," he said, "is not a person who is rich or powerful, but a contributor, a good human being. You can have all the money in the world, but if you aren't a good person, then what are you?" I have spent most of my childhood and adult years searching to refine others and myself in the spirit of my grandfather.

The path I've taken in this effort includes working and living with animals. This brings us to a fundamental question that needs to be examined: Can interacting with animals make us more compassionate and humane beings? For that matter, can working alongside animals make therapists better helpers? We also might ask how nonhumans help humans act with more integrity, empathy, and compassion. Those who have spent time with loving animals find these questions easy to answer. Paula Brownlee once stated, "To do good things in the world, first you must know who you are and what gives meaning in your life." For some of us, interacting with animals can be the first step to realizing and recognizing these values.

When I think of the afternoons spent with the children and my animals, I see similarities between the way I interact with my patients and the way the dogs, especially Puppy, also interacted. But I see significant differences between us. These differences are, in fact, where we can learn the most from our animals.

Golden retrievers are best known for their empathy and love. Jaime J. Sucher in his 1987 book entitled *Golden Retrievers* noted, "Your golden will love you for yourself. It gives its love unquestionably and completely; what greater devotion can anyone demand?" Just by their sheer presence and nature, goldens will stand by their friends. They seem to share a sense of unconditional regard and love that is, without a doubt, extremely durable. Using therapists' lingo, the term "empathy" defines a person's ability to understand from inside the perspective of the other person. It is being able to try to see the outcome through the eyes of others. Empathy incorporates compassion and care. Both of these features are part of the essence of a golden.

However, Puppy was not a typical golden. Perhaps her harsh beginning made her more sensitive to people, especially the vulnerable ones. She was patient with their needs and just sat by them to give them any support they needed. I can see Puppy, or for that matter any of my dogs, patiently waiting for a client to "get something out," to confide and unburden.

Michael, the father of a child with attention difficulties, sat in my office one afternoon confiding his fears that his child wouldn't amount to anything. His son struggled at school. He didn't fit in and was a challenge to his parents. Michael would do anything in his power to make things better, but knew he didn't have a magic wand to do so. The specific afternoon I am thinking about was devastating. He couldn't say anything positive and was feeling hopeless. Puppy sat next to Michael the entire visit as he poured out his misery. She looked into his eyes, seemingly trying to tell him that she heard his pain and wouldn't abandon him. Michael unconsciously began to stroke her head as he continued to talk. At one point he stopped our conversation and said, "Puppy, you are ok. Even as angry as I am, you make it easier to talk. Thanks for being here for me."

For a relationship to have any meaning it has to be built on trust. This is a dimension that both animals and people thrive on. When we put trust into someone, we know that person won't intentionally hurt us. Regrettably for Puppy, this wasn't true. As a young pup, she put her trust into a human who beat her. It took time for me to show her that not all humans are mean-spirited. In therapy, trust is established and built on the patient's belief that she/he will not be abandoned, no matter what is shared and revealed in the sessions.

Patience and a gentle approach are two other traits that are crucial in a therapeutic relationship. You cannot rush change. This is a weakness in some therapeutic relationships. I learned a long time ago that rushing an outcome can be devastating. I follow the old Chinese proverb that states: "Only when the mind is ready will the teacher come." We have to wait for someone to be ready for help, or at least be willing to accept it. While patience is a virtue that is worthwhile, a gentle approach nurtures and supports.

Throughout the years I have learned about people and the reality of therapy. I have had to learn that even when I have the passion in my heart to help a child make a change, there are times when the outcomes may not occur in the fashion or on the timetable I want. I've learned to be patient with life and appreciate the victories for what they're worth. Along with helping me be a more effective therapist, I have found my therapy animals have helped not only my patients, and their families, but also my outlook on building personal relationships.

Hart's Bark Insights: A Cuddle Is Worth a Thousand Words

You now know some of our "trade secrets," and they are simple and powerful. When you are feeling down or out of sorts, a tender touch can be as helpful as words. Sometimes verbalizing can aggravate the situation because you start to talk and find yourself, as a consequence, becoming more upset and stressed. On the other hand, some people, like Sarah, feel so insecure that they don't have the emotional energy or command of language to fight back or verbally express these feelings. They just hold everything in and feel so isolated.

When you are down, do whatever it takes to try and stay positive. It may take a while to heal, and unhealthy thoughts may take over. Believe us when we tell you that the negative thoughts will make things even worse. Some of you may find talking and being with others exactly what you need to edge yourself towards emotional recovery. Others may find solace in an animal. Whichever you choose, remember: Don't be afraid to give and receive a cuddle. We do it all the time. In fact, they are the best moments of our lives.

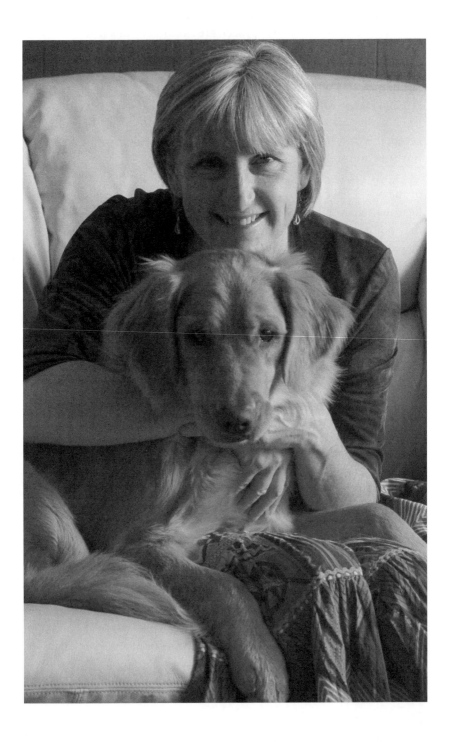

Fending Off Loneliness

Before class starts, Nicholas, a high school student, sits alone while others around him are talking and laughing. Craving connection with and attention from his peers, he jumps ungracefully into the nearest group's conversation. "Get lost! We aren't talking to you," is their response to him. He turns away, despondent and feeling increased alienation. "I am not invisible, I want to be seen," he thinks, "but they won't give me a chance. What's wrong with me?"

While most of us enjoy a wealth of human connections that make each day a tapestry of pleasant and appealing interactions, many people, like Nicholas, are disconnected from others. Sometimes loneliness goes hand-in-hand with a lack of confidence, and many times this lack of confidence reinforces alienation. Isolation and hopelessness can make us feel like inmates in a bleak prison. For these patients I look for opportunities for them to learn to open themselves up to the world and create friendships.

Because a life shared with friends is a more fulfilled one, friendships have always been very important to me. I began appreciating their value in my childhood when I witnessed several of my classmates becoming outcasts. They were often victims of verbal abuse and starved for attention. Even as a child, their pain was very evident to me. Like Nicholas, Philip, one of my childhood friends, never was accepted by most of our classmates. Unfortunately, he never knew how to handle verbal bullies and his reactions often led to confrontations.

I moved away during my high school years but would try to visit him whenever I could and stayed in touch until I left for college. Tragically, after years of feeling left out, Philip's life became one of almost total isolation. As result, his best friends were the athletes he watched on TV. In fact, he eventually was so obsessed with these "friends" that he wouldn't leave his house. Because Philip was treated poorly and didn't have help in coping with and learning the necessary skills to appropriately interact and build relationships, he became bitter. He could find no joy in life, and therefore no one could find joy in him. The life had been physically and emotionally beaten out of him.

In many ways my animals have helped me appreciate the fact that being surrounded by good company is worth its weight in gold. By nature, dogs are tremendously intuitive and sensitive animals, a condition society has a tendency to stifle in humans, favoring logic over our inner sense of well-being and balance. Dogs are especially good examples of how intuition and a willingness to open ourselves up emotionally can provide the basis for solid and long-lasting friendships. Dogs are not afraid to demonstrate their affection and will stand by you in good and bad times. In my personal life, all of my animals have acted as a strong source of companionship, and I cherish the time spent with my animals as I would any good friend. In fact, I am much more natural in front of my animals. To them it doesn't matter if it's a bad hair day or if I'm dressed to the nines. They see me in all my moods and through all my failures and successes, and what still impresses me is their tireless love and devotion.

My whole family loves to hang out with all the animals, including the birds. Snowflake loves to take walks with me. She just perches on my hand and is ready to go. When she gets excited, her crown begins to rise and she hums and lets out some screeching calls. She will even try to do summersaults as we walk. We're a real pair. She lets me know when she needs to get out of her cage with piercing caws and shrieks.

Taking the dogs for their excursions is another story altogether. Have you ever tried to walk three to four dogs at once, all at different physical levels and therefore different speeds? Sometimes I almost literally get torn apart. My arms get spread in different directions as the dogs attempt to drag me where they want to go. It is not that they are disobedient, but sometimes they are all just so excited to be out together that they forget I'm not an octopus. I regain control quickly once I let them know who is in charge of the reins. However, even after all these years, it never fails to surprise me how fun these walks can be. When at the park, I laugh as they romp through the fields and run back to me, almost trying to say, "Hurry up, slow-poke, you're missing everything." When they play, they amuse themselves with such exuberance that they make the event for me a pleasure as well as an adventure. On the other hand, we often just like sitting together quietly. Even in silence we are able to communicate very well—another characteristic of a sound relationship.

When Puppy was alive, she was attuned to my emotions. Whenever I was sad or a little edgy, she would make a point to just sit at my side. I often think it was her mission in life to console. Just having her next to me was sometimes all I needed to get out of my mood. I don't try to read and analyze my pets' actions, I just reap the benefit. I can recall coming home from a long day and not wanting to be around anyone. But when I opened the door, there stood Puppy, ready to rocket her way to me at the slightest encouragement. She sensed my needs but wouldn't push herself at me. Once I smiled and petted her a little, she went to work getting me to relax. She nuzzled her nose under my arm as if saying, "Snap out of it, Aubrey, life isn't that bad. You always have me."

But if these small, "everyday" experiences with Puppy were clues to the link between wellness and loneliness, recent months have cemented this idea, especially the benefit of animal companionship. As I mentioned in the last chapter, my wife, Nya, had been diagnosed with breast cancer. The family was devastated and we felt helpless as we watched Nya recover from her surgery. She tired more easily and at times it was difficult for her to be as upbeat as she usually is. I could see in her eyes that some days were just a battle to keep on going. I was totally frustrated and afraid. I did not know what to do and I was despondent when thinking of a future that did not include her.

Ask any woman who has survived breast cancer, and she will say there are ups and downs, and days that are utterly unbearable. Nya sometimes confides in me how angry she feels. She has always taken good care of herself (unlike me), and so when she was told she had cancer it was very hard to accept; and I felt lonely because she was also somewhat withdrawn from all of us. Over the months, she has tried to overcome her sense of discouragement, but I have learned to appreciate that the battle is day to day. Yet in this gloomy chapter of our lives, our newest addition to the family, Magic, proved she was correctly named. Often the dogs push the boundaries, and Magic is incredible at getting Nya out of a funk.

As you may recall, Magic joined our family when Nya was newly diagnosed, and over their short year together, they have leaned on each other for emotional support. Nya was like a mother chastising Magic when she got into the usual and unusual puppy pranks. Magic found herself in many jams with her mischievous ways and soft brown eyes— her mouth was often filled with anything from stuffed toys to tidbits of trash. Her favorite was bundled socks. This is when something mystifying happened; Nya did not respond to this mischievous behavior with rebuke. Instead, she just smiled and said, "Give it here." Magic responded with her tail going a mile a minute and pushing her wet nose against Nya. I teased her by saying, "Magic can do no wrong. She has you wrapped around her fingertips." Nya smiled and said, "She is no different than the rest, and you should talk. Look at how the others are pampered, especially Princess PJ." I smiled back, partially agreeing with her, but deep down I was aware of the unique kinship we both had with these animals. Magic could truly lessen Nya's sense of isolation, that feeling that many survivors of cancer have and that few people other than other survivors can understand. For a young dog, Magic had an amazing sense of concern for the tall human with kind eyes and an inviting smile.

Magic knows how to get past Nya's emotional armor. She is able to pick up on nonverbal clues that let her know when she's needed, even if an invitation isn't given. She just wanders over to Nya and nudges herself into her soul. Being a puppy, perhaps, has a lot to do with this. Magic is spontaneous and often acts without the reflection that comes with age and training. Like most golden retriever puppies, she is always on a "doggy" mission, which at times can be exhausting to watch. I wonder if that is why so many of us love to be around puppies. They bring out the best in most of us.

Nya is no different. Magic follows her around all day. When she wants attention, or when she feels Nya needs some attention, she asserts her presence. Magic can get away with urging more quickly than anyone I know. They appear to need each other and understand one another's unspoken needs. The other day when I came home Nya was in the family room sitting in a chair with Magic resting on the floor next to her. It was late afternoon, and I knew that Nya had spent most of it in the chair. After a few more minutes, Magic seemed to sense that Nya needed to get up and move. She stood on her hind legs and leaned into Nya; giving her one of those golden slobbery licks. Rather than resisting the attention, Nya began petting her, and then giggled and soft words started pouring out into Magic's soft furry ears, but Magic didn't just stop there.

Once she knew she had Nya's attention she moved in for the grand prize, one guaranteed to get Nya on her feet. She slid her front paws up on Nya's knees and before Nya could protest, Magic was in Nya's lap. Nya laughed. Magic had brought Nya out of her funk and back into the world of the living. Nya is recovering well, but the bond that grew out of this trying time has only gotten stronger. Magic is still Nya's constant companion and is never far behind with her stuffed toy in her mouth. Over the months I've often thought that I could learn something from dear old Magic. One of these times, when I'm in a jam with Nya, I'm either going to have Magic right next to me as a distraction or jump into her lap like Magic does. I have a feeling, though, that the former will work better.

What I'd like people to understand is that one or two friends of this caliber are all that is necessary to our well-being. Our measure as humans should not be how many people we know, but rather the quality of these relationships, and the first place we start learning about relationships is at home. How adults interact with one another illustrates to children the benefits and methods for building strong friendships.

I recently went home to Canada and had the opportunity to visit with various family members. I appreciate these special times because I can reflect on my past and relive many childhood memories. But when we are younger we may resent the time we spend with family because we'd rather be with friends. We don't always value family because part of the maturing process is this need to break away. Yet invariably we return. We return for a number of reasons, ones that we may not even consciously recognize.

On my last two days in Montreal, I spent several hours with my eldest aunt. She has been in poor health for quite a long time and has had difficulty with her mobility. She is now primarily homebound. Her condition worsened recently when she broke her hip and had to be hospitalized for seven months. She worried that she would never return home again. But she was able to move back a few months ago, with some social service help. Along with her continued poor physical health, she also is experiencing short-term memory loss and coping with the death of her husband. With all these changes she has a gloomy and demoralized outlook about her future.

Allowing people to age without dignity is shameful. But it is a sad reality for some who live their final years in imposed isolation, filled with loneliness. Unfortunately, my aunt was experiencing such a crisis. If left on her own, she would mope constantly and become self-destructive. "Look at what old age has done to me. I cannot move around and nobody picks up the phone to talk to me. I feel like a prisoner in my own home. I'm stuck in this small room and no one cares if I live or die." However, with a simple mention of the past, I could see a reignited sparkle in her eyes. Her entire demeanor changed as she said, "You remember, sweetheart, the good old days. Everyone would be here." She paused and looked up, almost trying to capture in her mind the happiness of yesteryear. "Your uncle, what a man. Don't you remember how he used to take you on Saturdays for your haircuts and then you would go get a hot dog and fries? He loved you and so did I."

What I sensed as we continued to talk, is how the reminiscing brought so much joy to her. She told me story after story. Their purpose, I know, was to emphasize that in the past her life had meaning and that she mattered. "Those were great days," she said in a trembling voice and with tears slipping down her cheeks.

This visit reinforced my appreciation of family as a continuing source of safety, comfort, and connection. Family also contributes to who we are. But I also realized that no matter what your age, family also remains a source of learning about life. The time spent with my aunt went by quickly as we spoke of years gone by. It was wonderful to see the sparkle in her eyes. She was in good spirits and a delightful companion, not because her condition and situation had changed, but rather because of our companionship. What she enjoys is being with others and talking, two things that she lacks on a daily basis but which have great impact on her emotional well-being.

It is sad to see where age sometimes leads us. In her early years, she was active and vibrant. Today her time is spent primarily in isolation, except when other family members look in on her, or volunteers come by to keep her company. The vibrancy of youth may die with age, but laughter, gossip, and the sounds of children laughing and playing can still be heard in the fabric of her walls as she reminisces of the "good old days."

Also during my visit, she spoke fondly of her daughter's dog, which recently passed away. For years, this pet was her official babysitter, and every morning, like the sunrise, Champagne hopped up onto her bed, gave her one quick lick, and then reclined next to her. This was the routine they celebrated for over seven years, until her recent passing. Champagne, like so many other animals in the world, filled the void of human contact. Companion pets are friends for seniors who would otherwise be isolated, and this was the relationship between Champagne and my aunt.

Yet seniors are not the only ones who may be isolated. Many people who have chronic illnesses feel both physically and emotionally isolated. Rachel, who is a native of San Francisco, comes to mind. Her life would have been empty without her furry and feathered friends. It is even more remarkable when you learn about her history and how she was unkind to animals as a child.

Today, Rachel adores her "kids," two dogs and a cockatiel—Tammy,

Maple, and Zeus respectively. Just how important these animals are to Rachel became evident after I learned more about her. Rachel shared with me her horrible, abusive childhood. Her parents called her "stupid" and "worthless" and physically beat her. As a result of this abuse, she developed emotional scars. Unfortunately, she found herself transferring her abuse to her pets. In looking back at her childhood, she explained, "I didn't know how to cope with the kind of love an animal gives to a human because my childhood was filled with anger and pain." Therefore she treated her animals as she had been treated. Her parents modeled a pattern of behaviors that she repeated because she knew no other way to express her emotions.

She continued this abusive pattern of behavior until one day she had a revelation:

> One day—it was a relatively good one—I became excited after hearing some good news. I remember whooping with joy and waving my arms. Then I caught sight of the dogs slinking out of the room. I followed them to a corner of the living room where they had stopped, cowering, and I had a shuddering flashback. I remembered one particular afternoon when my parents came home. They were very excited and animated, but my child's perception, based on my past experience, only saw the level of emotion and heard the raised voices as a danger signal. I ran to my room and crawled in bed, hoping to escape their attention. Then once more I was standing in my own house, and all in a moment, it just clicked. I realized that my abuse had to end. I was only repeating the pattern, hurting myself and my beloved animals.

From that day forward, she's never again hurt her animals, and they take care of her as much as she takes care of them. Whenever Rachel is sad, they are right by her side, giving her unconditional love. She says her life would be boring if it were not for them. "They are now my source of company, and whenever I can, I go walking with them at the park or on a beach. They give me the courage and energy to get out of bed and take pleasure in the world." Through her pets, she has been able to modify her behavior and learn the value of companionship. More importantly, this bond of friendship has helped Rachel extend her positive behavior toward the people around her and to establish human connections.

Abuse and aging are not the only way humans are isolated, but reading about and experiencing such cases is what led me to believe in the use of animals in my practice. At the start of my career I realized my clients would be victims of isolation and loneliness, but what I couldn't grasp fully was how difficult it would be to witness the suffering that they experienced.

Most of us have experienced loneliness at one time or another, whether self-imposed or inflicted upon us by others. Often this happens when we are removed from a familiar social network. Because our society is now more mobile, this kind of loneliness can happen frequently as we move from job to job or even across town. But it can also be a result of divorce or a death of a family member or a friend. No matter what the cause, the magical ingredient of friendship is missing, causing a sense of isolation, however temporary, from people with whom we feel connected.

This kind of loneliness, while uncomfortable, usually resolves itself when we reconnect or make new friends and acquaintances. But to ease this process, much can be learned from others in more extreme circumstances. Those who are bashful and shy, like Sarah, as we discussed in chapter 3, are in a distinct category of feeling alone. Their loneliness seems to be an outcome of their social anxieties and their discomfort in revealing themselves to others. These young people find themselves wanting to be invisible and develop a high degree of anxiety when they're around others. Sarah is a prime example of the tragedy that can befall us when we feel isolated. Luckily for Sarah, she met Hart, who helped her open up to life.

But if you add to isolation a physical challenge, diminished mental capacity, or learning disorder, then an individual's fear and anxiety may be significantly increased. My challenge as a therapist also is more complex when dealing with these added layers of defenses, fears, and anxiety while helping a child, a child like Paula. She was an eleven-year-old who was unhappy at home and at school, and her negative attitude was alienating others, including those who loved her best.

In our initial phone conversation, her mother told me that as hard as they tried to help her, change was difficult for Paula. As an infant, Paula's parents recognized that their daughter was developing more slowly than expected and started to have concerns. Eventually, when she entered school, her lag was even more prominent, and she was diagnosed as having a mild level of mental retardation. As the years passed, Paula developed behavioral problems and hyperactivity. At this time she had few friends and difficulty getting along with her family.

She spent much of her early elementary years behind a wall of silence, becoming a selective mute and refusing to talk or even interact with anyone. Although this refusal to speak reminded me of patients like Diane, Paula's refusal wasn't based only on fear, but also included anger directed at herself as well as others. But when others tried to be kind to her, she didn't reciprocate. Paula's only friend, according to her mother, was the family dog. They were happy together because Paula believed the dog had always accepted her as she was; therefore, she trusted the family pet, something she didn't allow herself to do with humans. Since I knew of her love of animals—especially dogs and horses—I made sure Puppy was around to work with her at our first session.

———

I walk out to the waiting room without Puppy. Paula answers my hello with a mumbled "Hi," her voice low—almost inaudible. I try to connect with her for two or three minutes but make little headway. I see visible signs of anger and frustration as she looks away, rolling her eyes and folding her arms across her chest. I judge quickly that the outcome of her first visit is going to depend on Puppy's ability to weave her magic spell with friendly eyes, a cold nose, and a wet tongue.

I know that her mother has used Puppy's presence to entice Paula's cooperation, and she is expecting to meet the dog. I realize more clearly that the anticipation of meeting Puppy is what has gotten her through my door. Surely, I think, Puppy will break the ice so that our afternoon will be productive.

I signal for Puppy and she enters the waiting room. She walks over and sits directly in front of Paula and puts her paw in the girl's lap. Instantly Paula's face lights up. Smiling broadly she says, "Oh, I love goldens!" She pets Puppy and then leans over and hugs the dog around the neck. Paula's whole manner visibly relaxes. With this connection made, Puppy, Paula, and I walk back to my office, where Paula continues interacting happily with Puppy—petting her, playing with her paws, and hugging her. Puppy continues to snuggle next to Paula, constantly prodding her for continued attention. After allowing this for a few minutes, I give Puppy a hand signal and she lies down next to Paula's chair. Now, I think, we are on our way.

Paula's reaction to Puppy is based on her experience with her own dog and Puppy's willingness to be a good companion. She trusts Puppy as she trusts her family pet. Therefore, her positive experience enables her to meet Puppy with greater confidence. With Puppy by her side, Paula began to talk to me.

"I just get so mad at everything. Nobody wants to be my friend."

When confessing her feelings, I observe that she speaks directly to Puppy—using her as a sounding board rather than me. But voicing her feelings has helped. Her body is relaxed and her tone of voice has softened. When our time is up, Puppy escorts Paula back to the waiting room to find her mother. Paula walks into the waiting room, her head up, smiling and with a confidence in her step that she rarely displays. By the mother's facial expression, I can tell that something good is also happening for this struggling parent.

Later her mother told me that when Paula returned home that evening she shared her experience about the "neat office" she had visited and her new friend, Puppy, the beautiful golden retriever. As the weeks passed, Paula's mother also told me that Paula looked forward to her biweekly sessions with Puppy and me—perhaps even more with Puppy than me, but this was okay. Puppy and I were a team, and in this case and at this time, Puppy was the stronger anchor for Paula. Feeling invisible and not being given a chance are two end results of alienation. The emotional cost of feeling left out is devastating because your sense of worth is diminished and you begin to second-guess your own value.

I incorporated a lot of "walking therapy" with Paula. Since she loved being with Puppy, the walks were not only natural, they were also the least threatening. Whenever we took Puppy for a walk in the park, Paula asked to hold the leash. To anyone watching, she looked like any enthusiastic twelve-year-old as she ran, laughing and bright-eyed, behind the prancing golden retriever. Taking a walk was a therapeutic tool for me, also. While concentrating on controlling the dog, Paula didn't filter or restrain her feelings, and she would speak more easily about the many issues she faced. Perhaps the greatest challenge she spoke about was alienation and not fitting in. In the months that followed, our sessions went well; in fact, they went better than I initially had hoped. Paula bonded with Puppy, and with Puppy at her side, she was able to relax and talk about the things we were working on. More and more she was willing to listen less defensively about her part in the alienation and to learn ways to make changes.

The hardest obstacle for Paula was to let go of the blame she placed on others, refusing any responsibility for her loneliness. This is a common reaction. If we can't or won't take responsibility for our actions and outlook on life, taking on the role of victim helps us rationalize our behavior and actions, and the blame then falls on those around us. But by doing so, we trap ourselves, just as Paula had done. A good illustration of how this works can be found in Charles Schultz's *Peanuts* comic strip.

Pig Pen walks around in a cloud of dirt that works as a form of isolation, keeping others at a distance. Similarly, blaming others results in a cloud of negative feelings. Although this cloud is invisible, people we encounter are aware of its presence through our actions, attitude, and words or, as with Paula, our silence. But Paula also had a little "Lucy" in her—so beware of the promise not to take the ball away, Charlie Brown!

Paula was defensive and never realized that she was projecting negativity. Once she recognized her part in reinforcing others' behavior, we could work on possible solutions. Our first goal was to help her act more pleasantly around others. Paula had a great smile, and when she let herself, she could project tremendous warmth. One afternoon I asked her about her difficulty expressing herself to the people around her, both at home and at school. I said, "Paula, you are so warm-hearted and kind to animals. Can you try acting that way with your family and others your age?"

Although I knew this would be a difficult first step, I also knew that without it Paula would be stranded in her isolation. She agreed to try, and we were now ready to work on reshaping her self-image and, more importantly, projecting this change to others. In our scheduled visits, we discussed sharing some of her good feelings toward animals with the people around her. With the help of Puppy, we even role played how she could demonstrate some generous gestures. It was quite a sight to watch Paula practice with both me and Puppy. She would talk politely and softly to Puppy to ask her things, and Puppy would respond back gently. Even when it was very apparent that Puppy didn't understand what Paula was asking for, she would stare back with her gentle eyes as if to tell Paula, "When you talk softly and kindly, I will do anything I can for you." Love is a great healer, and Puppy's love had begun to heal Paula's pain. Although Paula was initially reticent, she quickly began to realize that by sharing kindness at home she would receive kindness from others.

Her sense of social anxiety and her perceived incompetence made the battle of fitting in outside of home harder to overcome. I tried to break down some of her barriers and encouraged her to venture beyond her comfort zone and meet others. Although this may seem simple to someone without social challenges, for Paula this was traumatic. During our visits, we would choreograph assignments for her to practice. For example, we would plan out who she would talk to at school and the things she could talk about. I remember vividly discussing how she would have to sound positive and upbeat to the other girls to get a favorable response.

There we were, just the three of us: Paula, Puppy, and me. We practiced asking how the day was going and giving "girl" compliments to each other. Puppy would sit there patiently as we would say kind things about her. It was easier to do it with Puppy because she would not over-react, but rather would just sit there patiently as we practiced. Paula's goal was to put our exercises into practice and to update Puppy and me on her progress.

Some weeks later, she came into the office beaming with glowing reports on how she was doing. I could see her excitement as she debriefed us. There was such pride in her voice. Sometimes she would even write the incidents down in a journal so she wouldn't forget. I also could tell when the outcomes were not as favorable. It would be like pulling teeth to get her to tell the story. Luckily for us, her mom would get us started and fill in the holes that Paula would omit.

Our major goal was to expand Paula's social outlets beyond her family, her dog, and Puppy, and through these assignments, Paula's behavior began to improve at home and at school. Paula was receptive to the instruction and gradually became kinder at home. She was easier to get along with and there were fewer squabbles with her siblings.

However, a major setback occurred in October of 2000, when her good pal Puppy died. Paula had only known Puppy for a little over eight months, but she was extremely saddened to hear about Puppy's death. Although it was painful and hard, it was good for Paula to let the emotions out and to acknowledge her loss. Over the next month, many a tear was shed reminiscing about Puppy. In fact, about a month or so after Puppy died, Paula arrived with a ceramic cup she had made in Puppy's honor. I still have the mug proudly displayed next to a photo of Puppy. My friend may be gone, but her memory is still fresh in my mind, and sometimes I hear her walking down the hallway looking for a little attention.

Months later, when PJ began working in my office, Paula was thrilled. She really missed Puppy, and although Hart and Shrimp were fun, they were not golden retrievers. Once they became acquainted, Paula bonded well with PJ. In fact, I was surprised at how quickly and close an attachment they built. Paula loved PJ's innocence and found her gentleness and infant features irresistible. Like many children, Paula became attached to PJ because she liked to be needed. She began to see herself as PJ's elder, giving advice on life, such as on our walks, when she would often say, "Remember, PJ, that we have to look both ways before crossing the street."

Then one day she surprised me by asking, "Can PJ come to play at my house?" I told her that I would think about it and, before any action would be taken, I would see if her mother approved of the idea. Once the approval was given, I sat long and hard trying to figure out how I could incorporate her desire to be PJ's mentor into actual therapeutic goals. The psychologist in me believed that I could help Paula socially by challenging her to be a good pet-sitter with PJ. Over the next few sessions, we discussed what she would do when PJ came over and how she would have to share her attention with her other siblings and possibly neighbors on these short visits.

I stand outside my office waiting for PJ's return from her first "home visit." As the car pulls into the parking lot, I begin to laugh. Although Paula's dad is in the driver's seat, it is obvious who the VIP is. PJ, looking regal, sits in the front passenger seat, while the rest of the family is crammed into the back seat. The family spills out of the car while Paula proudly hands PJ's leash to me. Her mom says, "PJ seemed so comfortable sitting in the front seat we didn't want to disturb her."

PJ and Paula continued to be close, and Paula often asked me if she could "baby-sit" for PJ if I went away. In early June of 2002, the second year of Paula's therapy, I had plans to be gone for about a week. I brought up the idea of PJ's staying with Paula's family to her mom. It was Paula's last year of middle school, and after graduation she was going to be gone for most of the summer. She'd made progress in being kinder and more outspoken with her peers, and it seemed that our time together was ready to come to an end. Paula's mother and I agreed that having PJ stay at Paula's house would be a great way to enhance her sessions and might actually signal that the conclusion of her therapy was at hand.

Paula was thrilled with the chance. We spent several hours talking about the responsibilities of taking care of a dog, what she needed to know about PJ's routine and diet. Even more important, we talked at length about the fact that PJ looked up to Paula, so she needed to give PJ a lot of attention and act responsibly to not only PJ, but everyone around her.

Although PJ was apprehensive to leave me, she knew Paula and appeared very comfortable going to her house. I took over PJ's bed, lots of toys, and her favorite treats. Paula was going to be totally in charge. Immediately Paula's three siblings all wanted to have some time with their canine houseguest. This was a huge challenge for Paula, for although she had made a lot of progress in this area, she was reluctant to share PJ with anyone. This was one challenge she had to overcome. She needed to realize that we can share with others without feeling left out. She soon discovered their connection was solid enough for PJ to play with all of the children because it was clear that Paula was the person with whom PJ felt most comfortable. At night PJ was found tucked in under the blankets with Paula—something that doesn't happen even at home with my family.

Over the course of the week, Paula and PJ had a great time together. Some nights, the two stayed up late, listening to music in Paula's room and just hanging out. During the day, they took walks and played games outside—fetch and tug-of-war. Paula felt very confidant walking PJ, and as they walked around her neighborhood, lots of kids stopped Paula and asked about PJ. This was the perfect opportunity for Paula to connect with people in a new way, and she met the challenge with success.

After PJ's visit it was clear that Paula had turned a corner. She felt very good about herself. Paula's mom called to let me know that PJ's visit had been a great thing, not only for Paula, but also for the whole family. "PJ brought so much joy to the house. Paula made new friends on her walks with PJ, and, most importantly, you believed in her enough to trust her with the care of your special dog. It meant a lot to Paula."

That home visit was, indeed, Paula's graduation, both from middle school and therapy. I only saw her two more times after that. Her mom called me from time to time to let me know that Paula was adjusting quite well to her new school. She was still quiet, but she was making a tremendous effort to show her good side. She went to the football games and made a few friends. School was hard, but her attitude in doing her work was wonderful. She had learned not to give up on herself or others.

The last time I saw Paula was a few days before Christmas of that year. Late in the afternoon I unexpectedly found her in my waiting room. There she was, standing tall, with a beautiful smile. It took me a moment to even realize that it was Paula. She held a bucket of dog treats in her arms. I invited her in and watched as PJ greeted her with delight. Paula knelt and hugged PJ tightly. We sat together for about a half an hour that afternoon, Paula's arms never leaving PJ's neck. PJ reciprocated by cuddling closely to her and periodically giving her gentle licks. We talked about the things we'd done over the last two years—remembering our walks and talks, our memories of Puppy and what we loved about Puppy and PJ. Although I knew this was the last time I'd ever see

Paula, I had a strong suspicion that the essences of Puppy and PJ were going to be a part of Paula for a lifetime.

PJ rescued Paula from her glass house of isolation. Although more growth was needed, Paula now had the confidence and tools to venture beyond her self-imposed boundaries. She continues to be shy and soft-spoken, but she now makes an effort to be with others.

Paula's story had a more positive ending than some of the other children's lives that I have witnessed. Some of my patients experience loneliness not by choice, but rather because others see them as being odd or different. They become the target of ridicule for people who don't take the time to know them.

Many of us don't understand what it's like to feel lonely. Those of us who have no experience with such negative feelings are sheltered from confronting the unwelcome emotions that accompany the lack or loss of companionship, especially when this social isolation isn't by choice, as with the example of Nicholas.

While loneliness may be connected to and compounded by depression, each is a separate area of concern. It is evident that those who are depressed often remove themselves from the company of others, and those who are lonely want their alienation to be reduced and are driven to find others with whom to make a connection. Although this seems a contradiction, the two are linked, frequently working in a cyclical fashion. In many ways, the emotion of loneliness can be best described not as being alone, but rather of being without any definite and needed relationship. It's like sitting in a dark well with the sun and blue skies above and no way to get out of the well. We experience this to some extent each time we must interact with a new group. Millions of us have had the experience of going to a new church, new school, or convention without someone we know. We feel alone not so much because we arrive without a companion, although this is a contributing factor, but because we arrive without an anchor. We lack a tie, however tenuous, to the new group.

Another form of loneliness is found in people like Nicholas, who lack any emotional attachments. But again, we see a wide range of effects, and the causes can be from simply not knowing anyone in a group to not knowing how to interact appropriately with a group of strangers. Anyone who has worked for a company employing more than a few people has probably met someone suffering from this kind of loneliness. Perhaps you've worked with a person who, while on the job, is knowledgeable and efficient but cannot initiate or sustain water cooler chitchat. Or maybe you've worked with someone whose social skills are more in line with the class clown, for whom jokes and one-liners take the place of conversation. For these individuals, the emotional challenge isn't merely getting involved and meeting others; it is the formation of a meaningful relationship. We all need to establish at least one relationship that can serve as an anchor, whether in or away from the workplace.

For adolescents the workplace is, of course, school. But the two environments have a lot in common. Let's go back to Nicholas. I met Nicholas when he was seven and diagnosed with a language-processing disorder. Along with a learning disability, his greatest life challenge has been relating to his peers. It isn't that Nicholas is vindictive or hurtful, but rather he talks out of turn. When he joins into conversations, what he has to say doesn't seem to fit. On a smaller scale Nicholas's problem has probably occurred to many of us at least once in our lives, especially in new situations. So how do we establish a connection with others? What we need to realize is that this is a learned skill and is one good reason to afford our children opportunities to socialize at a young age.

Yet this is not always enough. When Nicholas was younger, his mother involved him in a number of social activities, but she was also in the habit of rescuing him when the social interactions became tricky. This worked well for a time because young children are more amenable, and, with guidance, some may be more willing to accept and tolerate those who are different. Unfortunately for Nicholas, his mother's taking and keeping control was more cumbersome as he became an adolescent because teens aren't as resilient and open.

Over the years, while visiting the office, Nicholas has established warm relationships with all of my animals, especially the dogs. He finds the office a safe haven where he can voice his concerns. Nicholas feels wanted when my gang of animals greets him warmly. In fact, he is disappointed when he arrives and the dogs have already left for the day.

Why can't the reception he receives from people be the same as he gets from the dogs? That's what he desires: going to a place where everyone is excited to see you. This deep longing for a sense of connection was one reason for the success of the TV show *Cheers,* which featured the motto, "where everybody knows your name." Cheers was the local bar that made people feel like they belonged. In fact, it was evident that many of the bar's patrons went there primarily so they could be connected to a community of friends. That is all that Nicholas wanted: nonjudgmental companionship and more intimate relationships within the community of his peers.

Life hasn't been easy for Nicholas, and he continues to feel isolated. But over the years, he has gotten involved more with others and is gradually becoming more accepted as he learns more appropriate ways to interact. He now is participating in some sports as well as taking on youth leadership roles. Yet he desperately wants the phone to ring and to be invited out by others, to be acknowledged and singled out as someone worth knowing. He continues to battle in this arena, but is making some strides in at least having more acquaintances. Establishing friendships and developing that circle of social support is a life goal that he, and many others, work towards.

Nicholas's and Paula's stories are by no means unique from many of the people I have experienced both professionally and personally. Although the loneliness experienced by younger clients seems excruciating, it's the loneliness I have observed in many of the young adults that hits home the most. Loneliness can be overwhelming, and some never find a way to overcome it.

Jonathan is about twenty-two years of age. Although he has accomplished more than his family could have imagined, he walks around feeling that his life is unfulfilled. He misses hanging out with peers and developing relationships. His sense of isolation makes him feel inadequate and unloved. What he longs for the most is to be accepted for who he is and to develop meaningful relationships, especially with women. Over the years, he has become more accepted, but he longs for the day that he has a girlfriend.

I met Jonathan when he was eight. Although now older than many of the clients I traditionally see, I continue to work with him, and he has had a remarkable relationship with PJ and the other dogs.

———

When he arrives, all the dogs clamor to get his attention. Even though I know he probably will not admit it, he gives PJ the most attention because he has a soft spot for golden retrievers. His face is relaxed and joyful as he sits on the floor surrounded by the dogs. PJ trots over to Jonathan, carrying a brush in her mouth, urging, actually begging, for a brushing. Jonathan has never refused her anything and today is no exception. It melts my heart to watch the two of them together. Jonathan's eyes are moist, and PJ squirms with pleasure as Jonathan brushes her.

In fact, when PJ had her first birthday party, Jonathan was very involved in its planning as well as supervising PJ at the event. It was great to see him feel comfortable around so many children, perhaps knowing better than anyone the emotional pain of loneliness that many of them were experiencing. Jonathan is a living testimony to conquering the fear of isolation. I wish I could have been in his shoes as he observed some of the children. What was he thinking? Did he feel sorry for them, or was he reminiscing about days that he wished he could forget? Was he happy for them, because they, at least, were invited to a party?

In fact, at the party one boy leaned over and hugged PJ and said, "Thanks, PJ, for inviting me. I promise I will invite you to my party, but it may be just the two of us. Hopefully, you'll like to swim." That boy still visits the office, and he looks forward to taking the "girls" for a walk. It is marvelous to watch the power of loving pets and the enduring influence they have on those who love them in return.

This reminds me of a young teen named Chloe. Chloe has spina bifida, and her parents, especially her father, encouraged her to get involved in outside activities. She was a Brownie, on a swim team and a cheerleading squad. However, as she grew older, she longed for a boyfriend. Although boys liked her as a friend, she longed for a more intimate relationship. After talking with her father she confided in me what she had finally admitted to him. "You know Dad; life isn't like a Disney film. You don't always get your 'knight in shinning armor.'" As she repeated this, she began to cry, and I confess my eyes weren't dry either. For those of us in mainstream society this discovery may sadden us for a while, but for young adults such as Chloe, it can be a crushing blow. She realized early in life that joys and disappointments were something to be shared, and without someone to share them with, joys can become disappointments, like a rose that dies before it can bloom.

Then there is Ron, who was eleven when I first met him. He came to see me because of his impulsivity as well as his severe learning difficulties. Just like the others we have spoken about, Ron's major life obstacle was his lack of social savoir-faire.

For Ron, my birds were what he found most interesting when he came to my office. At that time, not only did I have Tikvah in my office, but I also had a couple of peach-faced lovebirds as well as one cinnamon-colored cockatiel. Ron gravitated to the birds and was mesmerized. He often helped hand-feed the birds and was surprisingly gentle with these fragile creatures.

One fall afternoon he asked me how he could get a bird for himself. I called a local breeder and arranged for Ron to go by and purchase a small cockatiel. Ron was ecstatic. Once he had the bird at home he nurtured her with tremendous care and attention. The two of them became inseparable. Although Ron lacked human contact, his days and afternoons were filled with taking care of the little bird he named Buddy. Ron became so interested in birds that he built up his courage and joined a local bird club. After just a few weeks I could see the transformation, and during one session he defined his feelings: "Dr. Fine, the club is awesome. I learn a lot and the others in the club really talk to me. Me. They really like me."

Ron was so fascinated with the birds that he was willing to extend himself beyond his comfort zone. The result was that Ron met with success. He found a way to connect with others in a truly significant way. His new friends in the club encouraged him to breed cockatiels, and soon he was busy taking care of his own small aviary, thus opening a new chapter in his life. Although still shy and somewhat introverted, his strong interest in the birds, in something he loved and enjoyed, forged these new connections and involvement with others.

All of this reminds me of a story I heard many years ago, and I have now adapted and shared it the world over. In January of 1987, Elie Wiesel, the Nobel laureate, was the keynote speaker at the annual dinner for six hundred survivors of the Holocaust. At the reception he shared a moving story. When he was a child he came across a man carrying a bird in a cage as a birthday gift for a friend. "Does your friend like birds?" Wiesel asked. "I do not know," replied the man, "but come with me and see what happens." While walking towards the house, the boy asked many questions, all pertaining to why he would buy a bird for his friend. He waited eagerly at the home, but as the man was about to give his friend the gift, the friend smiled and requested that he open the cage and the windows in the room. The beautiful gift was setting the bird free. Once the request was granted, the man beamed with joy. There was no greater happiness for this man than setting another creature free.

Buddy had an equal but reverse effect on Ron. Buddy helped Ron set himself free and get beyond the confinements of his self-imposed cage—in this case, the four walls of his room. Finally, he was flying more freely in life and, most importantly, celebrating his flight. But it is also important to remember that anyone can feel lonely. Yet no matter how brief or enduring the time span, the impact is acute. Each day there are numerous ways we can show kindness to others—family, friends, coworkers, and even strangers—helping them lessen the loneliness. One such example is Sue and her pet partner.

Gleason, a yellow Labrador, and his owner, Sue, often visit patients in the local hospital. Sue extended her visits to include the maternity ward. On one such visit they met a young woman who had been ordered on bed rest for the last six weeks of her pregnancy. The woman, pregnant with her first child, developed a strong relationship with Gleason and Sue during the course of their biweekly visits. These were important to the young patient, especially since her husband was of little support and no other family members were available. One afternoon Sue stopped by the nurse's station to check on the mother-to-be and was told she had gone into labor, but the baby was in trouble.

The baby's heart rate was too low, and the doctors were considering an emergency C-section. When Sue and Gleason entered the room, Gleason jumped onto the bed and the young woman began stroking Gleason. After a few minutes, the monitor indicated that the baby's heart rate was climbing. As the patient continued to pet Gleason, the baby's rate continued to climb and gather strength, soon reaching the safe range. At the same time, Sue noticed that the woman's anxiety level decreased.

After two hours, Sue took Gleason home for lunch. But Sue had a strong feeling that she and Gleason should return to the hospital. Upon their arrival to the maternity ward, they discovered that the baby's heart rate had again plunged. Once more, Gleason was a source of companionship, helping the woman to relax during and between the contractions. As before, the baby's heart rate improved. Sue and Gleason stayed until the final stage of labor. An hour later, the baby was born, and, though premature, it was healthy and out of immediate danger.

Gleason's offer of companionship served as a source of strength and confidence-building. This, in turn, allowed the woman to relax and avoid a C-section, relieving not only her stress, but also the potentially dangerous stress level of the infant. Gleason may have intuitively sensed the mother's stress and need for companionship and answered that need eagerly and unselfishly.

Perhaps one of the most remarkable and beautiful outcomes I've witnessed with my patients was the transformation of a very awkward young boy, Steve, into a more confident, outgoing young man. Due to the severity of his issues, my professional relationship with Steve has been the longest I've had with any of the patients (entering the fifteenth year).

His mother, Brenda, was very concerned about her young son because he had seen various mental health providers, but little had changed. She thought that perhaps they had missed a crucial piece of what was going on with Steve. She had recognized that something was wrong very early in his life when she noticed that Steve's language wasn't developing within the norms. He had tantrums and was oddly obsessed with storms and the sounds of raindrops. Steve became so obsessed with the rain that he would stand motionless for long periods of time watching and listening to the rainfall. I diagnosed Steve with Asperger's syndrome, along with obsessive-compulsive disorder.

Like Ron, Steve was attracted to all of my birds. But he took exceptional interest in the smaller parrots I was trying to rehabilitate. He became especially interested in a small brilliant green-feathered dusky conure, and things were about to turn around for both Steve and Boomer.

Over the months, Boomer and Steve developed a terrific relationship. He eagerly looked forward to our therapy visits, and as with Paula, I was second on the billing. But that's okay. I want the children I see to learn to "fly" on their own. What I found was that Boomer's love and affectionate pecks calmed Steve when he was upset, and they developed such a strong bond that I allowed Steve, again like Paula, periodically to take Boomer home on "overnights" that eventually became visitations lasting several days. He was the first client I allowed to take home one of my small birds, and it was a step not taken lightly. Birds are much more fragile than dogs. But I believed that with proper preparation, taking care of my animals for short periods of time could become a valuable adjunct to my therapy, and how correct I was. It is difficult to understand how two completely different species can emotionally support one another, but one thing is true of all of us: We need someone or something in our lives to overcome depression and loneliness.

Of course, there were rules that Steve had to follow, including calling me on a daily basis to update me on how Boomer was doing. Steve loved taking care of her, and they became immediate friends. Steve stated, "I love Boomer. When I get home I know that someone is ready to see me. She's the calmest bird that I've ever met and she's real patient." Boomer's affection and positive therapeutic effect was a release valve for Steve. He knew she needed him, and as a result Steve became the nurturer rather than the nurtured. When Steve turned the corner, seeing Boomer as a friend, his outbursts were fewer and he often called to request a longer home visit with Boomer. "If I get really mad at home I try to stay calm and keep my temper down and that's when I like to take Boomer out just to hold her a while and calm me down."

Steve's deepening relationship with Boomer helped him better understand and control his emotions. As a result, both Steve and his mother reported improvements in his behavior and outlook. Even though Brenda initially had reservations—"He'll make a mess everywhere!"—She quickly saw a change in Steve. "One of the things that I guess every mother wants for her child is to be happy and to have self-esteem, and Boomer was something that made him happy. I feel that Steve is now going to have the chance to be happy as an adult. What more could I ask for? In the end I realized that any initial inconvenience was far outweighed by the benefits to Steve."

As Steve approached his eighteenth birthday, I looked back at his progress, and concluded his therapy was also nearing closure. I also realized that Boomer had been the magical ingredient. She had transformed Steve into a more stable and more sensitive young man. Boomer and Steve are matched perfectly. Within the limitations placed on their relationship, they had become inseparable. Seeing the relationship these two had, I came to a unique decision: What could I give this young man that would symbolize the importance of our relationship? How could I let him know how proud I was of him with all the changes he accomplished? The answer was easy. On Steve's eighteenth birthday I gave him Boomer, his green-feathered friend, who had taught him he had value. She showed him that a loving companion not only lessens feelings of isolation, but also can actually improve one's perspective. Although I was saddened to lose Boomer, I still know it was the right decision. I still can see Steve's eyes shining and hear the love in his voice as he took Boomer from me and whispered in her ear, "Boomer, you're with me now."

Boomer's new opportunity was the beginning of a new chapter in Steve's life. Like most of the clients I work with, I never really know where life may eventually lead them, but I do know that at this specific moment of their life, the emptiness that they had felt disappeared. We need to be grateful for those moments. I know they are. What Steve has learned through his companionship with Boomer has helped him grow into a fine young man, more independent than many would have fathomed.

Animals in general are more accepting of others and don't seem to require all the necessary social skills that are critical for human relationships. Is that why so many people have benefited from the love of their animals, especially those who are alienated and alone?

But animals can also feel lonely. Over the years I have learned to appreciate how my dogs need each others' company, and from my observations I've learned much about human beings' desire and need for friendship. Although humans believe they are "a dog's best friend," in reality a dog needs the companionship of another canine. PJ loves her human friends, but she loves being around her four-legged family members. Her truest joy is running and tussling with her adopted brother and sisters. The same can be said of humans. While pet companionship can be invaluable, we also need contact and connections to other humans.

Shrimp's Bark Insight

It was a typical Sunday morning in January. It was cool by southern California standards, but a beautiful day to get up and enjoy the outdoors. Every Sunday morning follows a similar routine: a leisurely breakfast and then it's off to one of our favorite walking trails. The other dogs go ballistic, sensing the change to the weekend routine and that a good, long walk is in the offing. They begin to romp all over the family room. Hart is doing the doggy rumba, shaking her behind like a Slinky toy. Magic, the youngest, usually leads the outpouring of enthusiasm by running to the open door to the garage and snatching her leash. She parades around the room, letting everyone know that she is going first. Miss Magic loves to flaunt her "puppy status." If she could, she'd like to be the lead dog, dragging the rest of us behind her.

But for me, today is a bad day. I'm struggling to get up. I want to go, though. I want to be with the family and the dogs. I can see by Aubrey's face that he's thinking hard about something. He looks at me and then the other dogs. Finally he said, "Shrimp, old boy, you're just not up to it. I promise to take you on a short walk this afternoon." They left me sitting by the door. I was dejected and felt a bit left out. Although I was disappointed, I was waiting in the same spot when they returned. I knew they would; I knew that my place in the family was secure and that Aubrey would keep his promise. Right when he got home, he kept his promise— just the boys out for a short stroll. We may have traveled only a short distance, but for me the walk was revitalizing. It meant the world to me.

My advice is to take a chance and make a new friend. My family has shown me that loving and being with others makes life richer and fuller. When we surround ourselves with people who care for us, we learn to care for others, and life's bumps are smoothed out. Just ask any of us, Hart, Magic, Snowflake or me.

83

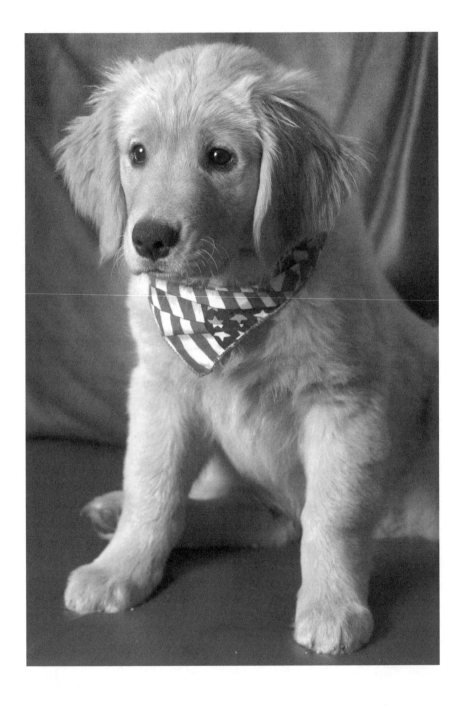

Do You Believe in Magic?

Excerpt from Ellen's dairy: "On the way to the first visit with Dr. Fine, I think we were all nervous. Sally was silent in the back seat of the car, clutching her baby doll. Her assistant and I were discussing ways to facilitate the visit and priming Sally as to what to expect. I had brought a camera along because Sally always liked to have pictures taken. These could be used as a reward for her. I have always known about her keen interest in animals. She isn't able to have a large animal in the group home, and recently she had overturned her bird's cage during a tantrum, luckily not hurting the animal. There was potential for problems."

"I'm 'eacher (teacher)," she says in a soft, quivering voice as she gazes into the on-looking eyes of Magic. I smile as I hear Sally proclaim her role with calm authority and remember my first meeting with this twelve-year-old, curly-headed girl. Only eight months have passed since then, and everyone working with Sally is pleased with her progress.

My contact for Sally was through Ellen, the case worker from the group home for children with developmental disabilities. I learned from Ellen that Sally had numerous behavioral challenges and was often openly hostile and physically aggressive. Options for Sally have been hard to find, and knowing of Sally's fondness for animals, we set up a first appointment.

In the months prior to meeting Sally, I had been training a young Magic to work with clients. She's showed signs of promise, but the training sessions are short because little Magic periodically needs to be a juvenile and can still lapse into puppy behavior. It isn't uncommon to find her, in her downtime, scavenging through the trash to find a tasty wrapper or dismantling one of her toys to get the squeaker out. But it is precisely this playfulness, along with her gentle manner, that makes her a lovable hit with my clients. I wondered if Magic's early experience nurturing Nya in her time of need has added a dimension to her sensitivity to others. Often she appears mature beyond her years; nevertheless, my gang still considers her the puppy in the house, and they let her know she has to pay her dues.

One of my clients suggested her name because he knew of my love for prestidigitation. He also felt the name was apt, especially if she could "magically" support children in therapy. I liked the name because I still use magic in my practice. It's a great icebreaker and an easy way to connect with clients. For a few moments, their minds are open to possibilities. This is what draws us all to the art of magic, and it is a way to teach children lessons of dexterity (physical and mental) while also impressing upon them the need for persistence in achieving a goal.

Thus, naming our newest canine member Magic was just perfect, for it represents two important dimensions in my life—a love of magic and a love of animals. The more I get to know this little one, the more amazing she seems. She continues to dazzle me with her sense of judgment and gentleness. At one moment, she is a calming cornerstone of compassion. At other times, she can be exhilarating to watch as she plays with an earnest zest for life. Being with Magic has convinced me that magic can be real, especially if we allow it to happen.

This brings us back to Sally, a child who needed to suspend her belief and be open to other possibilities. At our first meeting, she was sandwiched between Ellen and another staff member. I could feel the tension emanating off all three of them. Sally sat stone-faced, and her body was so rigid that I thought it might break with the smallest movement. Because I wanted to gauge her behavior, I met her without an animal companion. I sat down in a chair several feet away from them. Sally didn't speak much, but she mumbled the word "dogs." I spoke with her for a few moments, but Sally wasn't responsive. After another few minutes, I told her that I would go back and bring out PJ. She smiled. When I returned with PJ on a leash, her response wasn't what I expected. She immediately curled up into a ball and tried to cover herself. Her face grew pale, and her left hand went out as if to ward off an attack. She screeched, "No! No! No!" and spat at me. I had been cautioned this might happen, but it still surprised me, and I backed off quickly, leading PJ away.

Reassuring her that PJ was gentle and on a leash did not decrease Sally's anxiety, so I cued PJ to back farther away and lie down on the floor. That appeased Sally, and after a few moments, she relaxed and asked to see PJ. By the end of the morning, she had allowed PJ to come within petting distance, and Sally tapped the dog's head once or twice. Whenever I approached, however, she spat. Not exactly a perfect visit, but it was a beginning.

Later Ellen called to say all three of them were exhausted, but she thought additional sessions might be helpful. She then provided me with more critical background on Sally. She was uprooted and immigrated to the United States at age eight (about six years ago). She and her mother initially came to the United States only to visit, but during the visit her mother had gone into labor with Sally's brother and then applied for political asylum. Sally hasn't seen her father since.

After a short time, Sally's behaviors eroded. Her mom did not seem to understand that her daughter had a developmental disability. Sally had poor communication skills, and her reactive aggressive behaviors caused her mother to look for help. But Sally's aggression increased, and she started to randomly bite other children and spit at any adult that came near her when she was angry. Her limited language made matters worse, even though it was also apparent that she needed to express herself. Additionally, Ellen disclosed that Sally had experienced a traumatic event. She had possibly been abused.

After discussing incorporating the animals in her therapy, we resumed our visits a few weeks later. Sally entered the waiting room wearing a blue skirt and a white blouse, her curly hair pulled back with a cheerful barrette. She was more talkative that morning and remembered PJ's name. After talking for a few minutes and showing her my bearded dragon named Spikey, I told her that I would bring out PJ once again. Initially Sally had a similar reaction as on our first visit and moved away from the waiting PJ. Then, once again, she asked to pet PJ, but I wanted her to approach the dog this time. However, it wasn't going to be easy to get her to make the first move. As PJ sat patiently, Sally inched closer to her by moving to the end of the couch. I sat next to the leashed PJ, trying to coax Sally to get closer and to place her hand gently on PJ's head. "Sally, come over here," I urged. "PJ wants you to pet her." The staff also encouraged Sally to move closer.

Eventually, Sally moved to the edge of the couch, bravely stretched out her hand and gently petted PJ. I cued PJ to lie quite motionless so that she wouldn't startle Sally. We even got a soft brush for Sally to brush PJ's coat. It was a great start. Sally was leaning over the edge of the couch, just barely brushing PJ's fur. It was the first time I had seen her smile. She appeared not only content but also proud of herself. After a short while, we decided we were ready for our first walk. PJ was harnessed with two leashes, one for Sally and the other for me. We were escorted by the two staffers, who stayed very close to the three of us. We decided to take a short walk to increase the likelihood of a positive outcome.

Sally didn't speak too much during the walk, but her smiles told me she was happy. If PJ strayed even a little off Sally's planned course, however, she would get agitated. "No! No!" she said, as she almost dropped the leash. I quickly cued PJ to walk straighter, and Sally calmed down. Once we arrived back at the office, Sally fed PJ treats, which of course she gladly gobbled. A connection was brewing, but it was in a slow cooker.

Sally and I began to correspond with one another between our planned visits. She loved mail, and she enjoyed receiving notes from PJ. Ellen told me that Sally saved all the letters we sent her. Plastered on her walls were pictures of the dogs and the notes that she received. Sally also talked about our visits with anyone who would listen. The staff conveyed that she loved her office visits, although she didn't proclaim this to me in either word or action.

As the weeks passed, Sally's self-imposed barriers dropped, but that isn't to say things were much easier. Since Sally did well with PJ, I introduced her to Hart, to whom she took a strong liking. We also began to incorporate a few other activities. One afternoon we spent a portion of the time drawing pictures of the dogs and putting stickers on them. I made a photocopy for my file, which enthralled Sally. "Make copy," she insisted. Then "I do it" followed as she requested permission to press the start button. She was insistent that we make several copies of all her drawings. If she'd had her wish, we would have used a ream of paper to copy that one picture. Eventually, with the help of her staff, she was led out of the room.

Although we were making progress, she still needed a lot of encouragement to get closer to the dogs. Once she was next to them, however, she seemed to relax. The same held true for our walks. She loved going on them, but periodically some of her resistant behaviors reappeared.

Unfortunately, my early visits with Sally were often interrupted by scheduling difficulties at the group home, and this was an obstacle. When we didn't meet on a regular basis, we had to start all over. Her anxiety about the animals returned, yet she had a strong desire to be with them. I talked with Ellen about this, and we both agreed that a more consistent schedule would help Sally become more comfortable. We wanted not only to help Sally overcome these fears, but also to enable her use of words rather than act out aggressively in frustration. For example, when Sally felt anxious, her first response was either to spit or to step back and cover herself with her arms.

Reflecting on my initial work with Sally, I thought it would be a good idea to incorporate Magic because she was a little smaller than PJ. Although PJ is very gentle, Magic can be a bit more timid. I had been working quite hard with Magic over the past several months and believed that she was ready to work with Sally.

When Sally arrived that Friday morning, I told her that she would be working with Magic. Initially she kept asking, "Where's PJ and Hart?" Because I wanted to show a spark of interest in Sally, I let her know that Magic was a puppy and that she would need all the help that Sally could give her. Sally needed to help Magic become more comfortable and unafraid. I kept repeating her role as Magic's teacher, and eventually she grew excited at the prospect.

I called to Magic, and when we could hear her approach down the hallway, Sally leaned forward for a glimpse. On a typical visit, it usually took a few minutes for Sally to work up her courage to approach the dogs. Today was different. When Magic entered the foyer, I cued her to lie down; she looked baffled but complied. I then turned toward Sally and reminded her that Magic was new to this and needed Sally to be gentle and kind. Because of my previous experience with Sally, I was surprised when she followed my instructions. She sat on the floor next to Magic and began to pet her. This was a first. She didn't seem uncomfortable at all.

Although there was some distance between them, Sally looked more at ease. She asked for a brush and began to brush Magic's fur. She was so engrossed in taking care of Magic that her comfort level increased. She wasn't as guarded with Magic and was even playful. She put her hand next to Magic's paw and said, "Slap me five, Magic." Then she giggled when I helped Magic comply. I was impressed with both of them. Next, and without any hesitation, Sally rested her head on Magic's tummy. This was the last thing I had expected. After a few moments, Sally gently kissed Magic's face. This was another first for Sally. Finally, I thought, she was opening up. Magic reciprocated by turning her face slowly toward Sally and licking her face. After a few moments, we went for a walk around the block.

Sally was in the mood to talk. She told me about school and some of her classmates. She also started to sing a song. Sally was still interested in the other dogs and asked several questions about them. "How is Hart? Where is PJ? When I see them, can I give them a treat?" Today it was finally clear that Sally was becoming more responsive to both me and the dogs. While we were walking I wanted to make sure that Sally continued to focus her undivided attention on Magic. I continually reminded her to let Magic know that she was doing a good job. The prompt was all Sally needed to refocus.

Sally stopped walking and gazed into Magic's eyes. "Good job. Good job, Magic!" she said. She then looked at me and said, "Give her treat" as she held out her hand. Just hearing those words were music to my ears, not to mention the puppy's. Sally took a few morsels of a biscuit and fed them to the waiting Magic. Both seemed very pleased with the outcome (Sally also got her snack). As we walked, Sally stopped several times and told Magic to either sit or to stop, speaking calmly and clearly.

I was impressed with both of them that early Friday morning. Sally was taking to heart her new role as a teacher, and Magic was a star student. Perhaps for the first time in her life, Sally was put in a role where others expected her to act responsibly. At least on this day, taking on the extra duties seemed to be a good idea. Sally worked hard that morning. Her comfort level with Magic was much higher than with the other dogs, although she constantly talked about PJ and Hart. Even when frustrated, she was learning to communicate verbally and appropriately. She was more confident and allowed herself to make mistakes. She was more accepting of her own erratic movements and trusted the dogs.

The sessions with Magic continued, and the bond between the two of them strengthened with each visit. She reminded me at the start of our sessions that she was "the 'eacher." Sally's new confidence was also evident at the group home. Ellen said the dogs were Sally's favorite topic. Whenever she returned home, she told anyone who'd listen about the

"the girls" at Dr. Fine's office. The staff used this new interest to defuse potential conflicts, reminding Sally that she was Magic's role model. Additionally, Sally showed an interest in art and enjoyed adding her drawings of the dogs to her wall of letters and photos.

Most importantly, Sally has started focusing her concern on the dogs rather than herself. On a recent visit, Sally saw PJ's paw was bandaged. I explained that she had a broken nail and that the bandage helped prevent infection. Through our session Sally kept asking, "Will she be okay?" I was later told that when she returned home, she drew several pictures of PJ that illustrated her bandaged paw. When Sally returned to the office, before I could say a word, she asked, "How is PJ doing?" and she was reluctant to start our session until she saw for herself that PJ was better. Looking right into PJ's eyes, she asked in a serious tone, "You okay PJ? Where's your bandage?" Sally then took out a picture she'd made of the dog's injured paw. Before PJ left the room, Sally gave her a big hug.

At this writing, Magic and Sally have worked together for seven months. PJ and Hart still get a chance to visit with Sally, but her direct copilot in therapy is darling Magic. Pairing the two of them has been powerful. In retrospect, placing Sally in the role of Magic's teacher was a great idea. I will never forget her smile at the news of her supporting role in Magic's training.

During these last months, one of her jobs has been to help Magic ignore distractions. Although this training is helpful for Magic, indirectly I am more interested in helping Sally with this problem. One of Sally's greatest challenges has been her strong curiosity towards babies being pushed in strollers. Whenever she sees babies in strollers, she gets unusually distracted and at times agitated. Our first few training sessions went well, but they didn't include a direct challenge for Sally. So prior to a visit, I placed a baby stroller and doll in the parking lot. After greeting Magic and brushing her, we headed out for our walk.

Once we entered the parking lot, she noticed the stroller. There was an immediate change in her behavior. She was agitated and distracted. I walked close to her and said, "Sally, walk away from the stroller. Remember you're the teacher and Magic needs help with this distraction." This simple redirection was all it took to focus Sally back into her task. She lowered her voice and said to Magic, "No Magic. Walk away. Walk away." Magic complied, walking around the baby carriage. Sally's look of pride told me she was happy that Magic had listened and that she, too, had done well. "Good dog, Magic!" she exclaimed as she gave the dog a treat. By the end of the walk both Sally and Magic were full of pride and were awaiting their earned special treats. Magic gobbled up her jerky, while Sally held on to her bag of trail mix.

By the end of October, I felt Sally deserved a larger reward for her progress and promised that on her next visit she'd receive a surprise. Just before the session, I picked up a pizza and some drinks. When Sally arrived, she was very excited. She remembered our plans and was ready to party. She brought along a stack of pictures of her family living in her old country and in the United States to show me. She introduced me to all the people in the pictures, as if she wanted me to know more about her life outside this office. After talking for ten or fifteen minutes, we enjoyed the pizza and drinks. Sally was an excellent guest and thanked me for arranging this special event.

The highlight of the morning, however, was when Magic paraded out wearing her Halloween clown costume, which was bright yellow with blue and red dots. Sally shrieked and giggled when she saw her. She immediately told Magic that she was going out as a go-go dancer. "I show you next time I come. I bring picture," she told her. In the middle of the sentence, Sally flopped onto the floor next to Magic and began to brush and pet her. She now was so comfortable with the dog that she kissed her on the head. I told Sally that after we took a walk, we had a few more surprises for her. Sally seemed excited about the gifts but was glad about the walk. She was extremely talkative and even showed a sense of humor. She giggled and gave Magic lots of praise and loving. But what was most memorable was the return to the office.

Sally went to the van with the staff members while Magic and I went into the office to gather gifts. I returned to the van with a small bundle of candy while Magic followed, cradling in her mouth a masked and hooded Halloween teddy bear. Sally beamed with joy. I was equally pleased to see that Magic was willing to relinquish the toy to Sally. She was surprised and it took her a moment to comprehend the gifts were just for her. After she said "thank you" to us, we turned to walk back to the office. But Sally called us back. She said she needed to come out and give us a hug. She left that morning knowing she was accepted for who she was. She knew we cared for her and that the feelings were mutual. Was today a new beginning? Was there a little magic in the air? All I know is that after a short visit that morning Sally left feeling like a new person. Magic had done her job. But what would all of Sally's tomorrows bring?

Ellen has continued to keep an ongoing diary of Sally's progress after each of our visits. Let's take a quick glimpse at what she has recently written.

Each visit her autonomic reaction has decreased – initially her hand was ice cold and pulse rapid through the walk until returning to the parking lot. Her eyes would dart around, glassy, and huge. She looked petrified. She had limited eye contact with both Dr. Fine and any of the dogs she walked. She looked hyper-vigilant and easily distracted by all the sights and sounds of the environment, looking past the dogs instead of at them. Now she is so much more relaxed with everything! There has been a steady increase in her language abilities. I have been impressed with her ability to identify some emotions and state them to us as she walks. No longer does she spit or lose attention immediately upon encountering a new adult. Now she relates to adults much better. Sally seems to have more self-awareness. She seems more content when she leaves. She does not fall asleep after visits (i.e., they do not seem so emotionally exhausting anymore; they are more therapeutic).

She seems to want to talk about the visits, Dr. Fine, and the dogs when she is at home. She doesn't seem to want to disappoint the dogs. She recognizes all the dogs in pictures. Recently, I gave her a beanie toy dog that was a golden retriever, and she immediately called it PJ. We no longer have to take pictures during visits because she is more interested in what we are doing. She is excited and anticipates coming. She knows the route, and when I am not driving, she tells the other driver where to turn. She is making progress and that is all that counts.

The last visit took the cake. Instead of interacting with the dogs right away, Sally wrote a letter to Magic with the help of Dr. Fine. It was remarkable! I have never heard Sally talk so much. She was so excited to do this. One statement in the letter put into words why her relationship with the dogs, and especially Magic, is so meaningful to her. She writes, "Thank you, Magic. You make me feel like a good girl; I love you." I guess magic can be real, especially if you believe in it. I am a believer now!

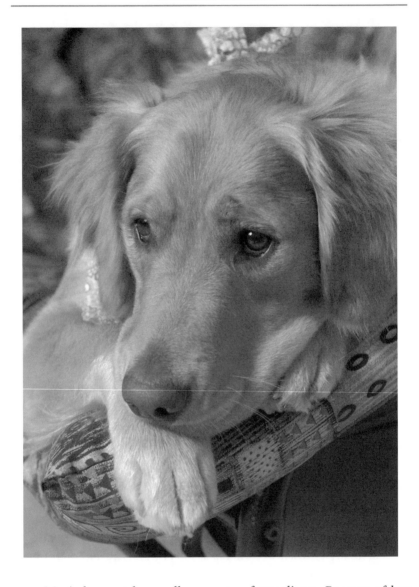

Magic has cast her spell on many of my clients. Because of her youthfulness, it has been quite easy to involve a few of the clients in her training. Again, all I can say is that I have been in awe of the outcomes. Over her short life, not only has she cast her spell on Sally, but also she has worked at three high schools, even helping a senior student with a project.

As I mentioned before, Magic's training had started prior to our meeting Sally, when she was five months old. I had several children who had asked about helping her, but one of my clients was determined to get involved. Scarlet, a tenth grader I have known for about eight years, has interacted with all my animals. We have a good relationship, and, as with many of my clients, a highlight is our interactions with the animals. Although she has made significant social progress over the years, life continues to be difficult for Scarlet. Challenges both at school and at home linger. Her impulsive reactions and her social immaturity cause difficulties with peers. Her difficulty in processing information and working at a slow pace makes completing her schoolwork arduous. However, what Scarlet has going for her is a supportive, loving family and a willingness to accept support and guidance.

Scarlet was the most persistent of all my clients in asking if she could help with Magic's training. Once I agreed that it would be a good idea, we spent some time in our sessions discussing her role in the training and the importance of her taking on this role with responsibility and maturity. We eventually decided (as part of her therapy) that we would meet once a week, so that she could accompany Magic and me to puppy training classes at a local park. The class started at 8:00 a.m. and Scarlet always arrived well ahead of me.

But the lessons were not going to be as simple as she expected. At first, Scarlet needed a lot of supervision because, upon seeing Magic, she'd be so excited and animated that the puppy's behavior also escalated. For example, during the first few lessons both of them behaved inconsistently. One day Magic took off to chase a candy wrapper blowing across the grass, and Scarlet dashed off after her. She was as excited as Magic, laughing and egging the dog on. Scarlet needed to realize that her behavior influenced Magic's. Therefore, she had to be the role model, since Magic was to look to her for guidance on what is acceptable behavior for successful socialization.

For eight Saturdays, Scarlet met Magic at the park. In addition, she also came by the office once or twice a week to practice. In spite of a few early sidetracks, Scarlet developed into a caring and diligent teacher.

One of the therapeutic techniques that I incorporated into Scarlet's therapy was the use of a reflective diary. In thinking about her work with Magic, I wanted Scarlet to recognize that she could be a giver and that she could make a difference in someone's life. This is a brief glimpse at her reflection: Scarlet titles this reflection "There's a little Magic in Magic."

My time with Magic has been amazing. The first day that I saw Magic at Dr. Fine's office, I instantly bee-lined right over to her. She was so adorable, mischievous, energetic and play-ful. I swear, Dr. Fine had to pry Magic from my arms. One day when we were talking, Dr. Fine told me that he was going to train Magic, and I asked him if I could help him. You could see him thinking about it, and he eventually told me that he thought it would be a good idea. A few months later, I brought up the subject about when I could start training her, and we decided we would start once school ended, in the beginning of June. I was so bubbly and happy.

What Magic taught me was amazing. One of the many things that she showed me was to have patience. Dr. Fine would tell me that I needed to have patience, and to keep prac-ticing and practicing. Just because Magic sat down on our first attempt doesn't mean that she got it. I guess it's safe to say that I was a bit eager to try new things/tricks with Magic. Even though I had my fair amount of frustration, and I'm sure that Magic probably did too, I still had fun.

Magic taught me about responsibility. Boy-o-boy, when-ever Magic wanted to play/fool around with me at training class, I would jump at the opportunity. Sometimes I would get carried away, but eventually I would quickly get back up and refocus my attention. Over the time of the class, I got better at not fooling around when I was not supposed to.

My mom pointed something out to me the other day. She asked me how I liked being a parent. Me, of course, being dumbfounded, didn't know what she meant. Mom said that I was sort of like a "parent" and that Magic was my "kid." How did I like it when Magic ignored what I was saying? So, in a way, I guess you could say that I learned responsibility through being a "parent" to Magic. This is an experience I will never forget.

I also used this technique with Stuart, also a high school student. Stuart is soft-spoken and has a good sense of humor. However, his chal-lenge was a lack of follow-through in his school work and periodically making some poor social choices. Even though Magic and Stuart do not now work together as often, they forged a strong connection, and Magic is always excited whenever Stuart has an appointment. Even if a month has passed, she greets him with enthusiasm and frequently comes into the room carrying her leash in her mouth. Again, I'll let the diary entry speak. Like Scarlet's, his words express best the power of his relationship with Magic.

> *All people make mistakes. Some are simple ones that only re-quire an apology, while others require much more. In any case, all mistakes are bad, but what is more important is what you can learn from them.*
>
> *Unfortunately, I have recently made one of those mistakes that were much bigger than normal. Back almost a year ago while I was at my old school I made a major mistake. It was during lunch and I was feeling kind of bored. I came up with this stupid idea to make a prank phone call to the police on my cell phone. I didn't think they could find out it was me. It wasn't until the middle of my next period that I was called to the office into the dean's office. When I arrived there, I had to wait for a short period of time. I started to get sick to my stom-ach. When I finally got in there I found myself facing not only the dean but an officer as well. To make the situation worse, I had denied the fact that I was the one who made the phone call. I denied it all the way up to the polygraph test, which of course I failed.*
>
> *After this all happened, and my parents found out, my life seemed pretty horrible not only at home but at school as well. At home I was grounded from everything, and when the school had been notified that I had made the call, they consid-ered expelling me. If it had not been for my dad's help, I would have been expelled.*
>
> *Even though I was never expelled, I was still given com-munity service hours to complete. That is where my real re-lationship with little Magic begins. I had seen her in a few of my office visits, and I always enjoyed hanging out with the animals. When I first brought up the idea of doing my service hours under Dr. Fine's supervision I didn't know what to ex-pect. At first I imagined that the experience would be boring, almost a punishment for my poor choice. I thought all I would be doing is just walking the dogs around the block. But after the first two times, I started to train Magic. Dr. Fine went over some basic commands and showed me how to work with her. I grew to liking these hours because it was a time for me to re-*

lax and be with one of my favorite animals. This was a great experience that came from my mistake.

Magic still needed some training when I began to work with her. Although she knew various commands, she didn't always follow them. She was also somewhat energetic and playful and would use any excuse to raise some havoc (I got a kick out of that). When we started the training, she would always try to get back inside the office. She seemed to be confused about why she was outside working while the other dogs were relaxing inside. What excited me the most is that over time she seemed to look forward to seeing me. When I would come in to get her, she would get excited and start to jump around. Like Magic, I had also grown to liking her more and more each time I saw her. Though training her could get tough from time to time, I always walked away feeling as if we accomplished something, especially when she was so affectionate while I was there. It was a good feeling to know she was learning and getting what I was teaching her. It was like the feeling you get when doing great on an exam or some other project.

For example, I tried to get her to shake hands. At first, this was really tough. All she wanted to do was sniff the ground. After trying many different ways with lots of treats, I discovered that when I gently blew on her nose, she lifted her paw. You should have seen me. I was so excited. I felt great! I felt like jumping up for joy. From that day on she seemed to get the hang of it.

Over a few months, I would work with Magic twice a week. Once she got to know me, she got extremely excited when I came over to the office. She would forget all her obedience training and jump up and try to give me a hug. Her tail wagged totally out of control. You really knew she was happy to see you. On the other hand, PJ looked jealous and eventually would butt in to get her hugs. I knew then how much I meant to both of them. Dogs are my favorite animals. You can tell they want to be around you because they show their joy when they see you. Their tails are wagging and their entire bodies shake!

Working with the dogs gave me a sense of accomplishment and a feeling of being worthwhile. It isn't something that is easily explained because the experience is personal and pri-

vate. I have learned in my own life that whenever you are with any dog, you always feel somewhat safe and happy. The experience of hanging out with them just makes you have a good feeling all over because of their actions and the kindness they give in return. That is the greatest feeling that I got from the experience of training and playing with her. I also got some quiet time. When we went for our walks, it gave me time to think of the past, of what I had done, and what has happened since. Most of the time, I thought about my future and what I needed to do to not repeat the same mistake.

Although I started this experience as a repayment for what I did wrong, I will always look at my time with Magic as a blessing. Even if things were not working out, I could always look down and see a dog's face that would pull me out of that mood. I now believe that I understand what Dr. Fine meant when he said, "Dogs leave paw prints on our hearts." There were evenings when our time was almost up and I was about to leave. Magic would try to make me stay by grabbing onto the leash with her mouth and jerk and pull it crazily like she wanted to play tug-of-war.

I feel very grateful for my experience with Magic and PJ. They allowed me to do some good. I now feel better about myself. The service hours weren't a punishment at all, but a lesson that I could learn from. Luckily I worked with a dog that put her loving spell on me. I guess she really does have a little "magic" in her.

Many magicians are often asked the question, How are the tricks really done? Or, Do you know how Copperfield made the Statue of Liberty disappear? Or, How does David Blaine, the outstanding street magician, levitate himself while performing in the crowd? My typical response is to concur with the questioner's tone of awe. "Wow! Wasn't it great?" But sometimes this is not enough; the questioner wants the specifics, the "tricks of the trade." Here I fall back on the magician's oath—never reveal the secret as to how the illusion works. However, I will let you in on this part of the secret: Magic is a contract between the illusionist and the audience. The greatest part of any magic trick is the audience's willingness to believe, even for a moment, that anything can happen. That is what I love the most about illusions. We suspend our belief and allow the performer to guide us, to redirect our attention. If we concern ourselves with only the technicalities, we miss out on the fun—the idea that, indeed, anything is possible if only we believe.

Kevin James is a brilliant artist who performs magic all over the world. He has many outstanding routines, one of my favorites, which I have performed a few times, is when he makes snow. Kevin performs this illusion with panache. The audience listens to him talk about sharing the miracle of snow with a child. We watch him tear some pieces of white tissue and drop all the torn pieces into a glass partially filled with water. We then watch him fish the wet pieces of tissue out the glass with his wand and wring out the excess water. As he continues to talk, he starts rubbing the pieces of wet tissue in his hands, and suddenly, the pieces of paper begin to fly into the air and flutter downward, giving the appearance of a snowstorm. The illusion is beautiful. For a few moments the audience, seated in a warm and comfortable theater, is treated to a cascade of delicate snowflakes. No matter how often I see it performed, it takes my breath away, and I'm transfixed for a few moments.

Sally's, Stuart's, and Scarlet's lives were transformed because they had the courage to suspend their belief, to think about a new way of looking at the world.

Magic's Bark Insight

We all need to believe in magic. We need to allow the unexpected to happen and believe that good can come from it. In every child, as indeed in every adult, there is a need to believe in the impossible. In all of us, there is a yearning for fantasy and wonder and make-believe. It is to this heartfelt yearning that magicians direct their appeal. When we see snowflakes appear as if by magic on stage, or when a silver ball floats around the performer; when we enjoy the illusion of a lady changing from a red to a yellow dress, or even the mystery of a vanishing elephant—at such times our daily burdens melt away, we are lifted out of ourselves, and for a few minutes, at least, we experience contentment and bliss.

Some say I perform magic. But all I really do is help the children believe in the possibilities of miracles, just as the magician does with his audience. Every day we can explore the magic in our lives if we yearn to, but we don't need to know the why or how of this magic to enjoy the benefits. Sometimes just the magic of loving and caring for someone, of being more

100

open to another's love, can make the difference. However, it's not always feelings that bring about action; rather, action can induce the feeling. So we shouldn't be afraid or too proud to offer our hand or accept another's. It's the best way to find a little magic when least expected.

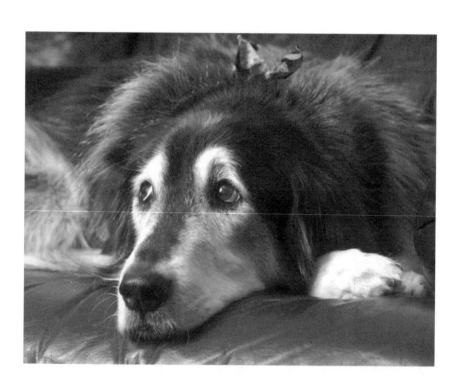

Giving and Accepting a Second Chance

Mending a Broken Soul: The Lesson of Giving

I'm sitting, listening to an animated Chad. "Sometimes, Dr. Fine, Polly climbs off her perch all by herself and wanders around the house 'til she finds me." I can hear in his telling of these events that Chad's relationship is still evolving. As I continue to listen, I'm encouraged not only by how he talks of Polly, but also by the evidence that he's learning from her. "She chewed up my favorite baseball cards. At first I was angry, but then I realized she didn't mean to. Polly just doesn't know any better. Even though she makes a mistake, I still love her."

———

This acknowledgment is an important step in Chad's progress. His relationship with Polly is a model he can build on. In learning to forgive Polly, he is also learning to forgive himself. He's beginning to understand that we can like ourselves, even our flaws, because no one is perfect and because we have to recognize our faults as well as our strengths. Moreover, Chad is learning that it's rarely too late to make a fresh start.

In my practice I see all types of children with varying degrees of need; they are troubled, abused, or have physical and emotional challenges. As you've read so far, a number of these children have multiple challenges that are interlocked and frequently feed off each other. Some of these children have locked themselves away emotionally, some have the desire to change but lack the tools, and still others, like Chad, find it easier to give in and give up—accepting what others think to be true.

Chad's needs were great, both academically and socially. Unfortunately, he had become a victim of his own failures (giving up) as well as buying into what others told him he was (giving in). What Chad needed was a "re-do," a way to view his life as having meaning while also accepting his limitations. This is where Polly's serendipitous appearance in both our lives made all the difference.

Over the years a local veterinarian has called on me to rescue animals. Most often this is a temporary arrangement I take on gladly until the animal is trained, rehabilitated from injury, or recovered from illness enough to find a permanent home. This was the case with Polly, a dusky conure with green and orange feathers. Polly was born with a deformed claw and wasn't getting the proper nourishment and attention from her mother. Besides her failure to thrive, the breeder was concerned that the bird would go unsold if she couldn't learn to perch, bad claw or not.

Polly was trusting, gentle, and still young enough to require handfeeding. Because of her age and frequent need for meals, I took Polly to my office each day, placing her small cage next to me. Almost simultaneously I began to see Chad, and after a feeding, he would offer to hold and pet her, and she seemed to enjoy this contact. She would waddle over to Chad's outstretched hand and wait to be lifted. Chad was fascinated with Polly's determination to move about despite the bad claw. "She's a fighter, Dr. Fine. She hasn't given up, has she?"

In time, I began to teach Polly how to perch using double-sided tape to help her grasp more effectively. I also lowered the perch so that if she fell she wouldn't hurt herself. As I went through the process, I could see Chad out of the corner of my eye. His focus was on Polly. I could sense a tension in his body as I moved my hand from supporting the bird. The question hung heavy in the air: Could she hang on? When she managed for a few seconds, I heard a rush of air escape Chad. Like me, he'd been holding his breath in anticipation. After this exercise Chad asked if he could stay beyond his session to help Polly learn. Since he was my last appointment of the day, it was arranged with his mother and became a routine for both of us. With the aid of the tape, Polly was able to train and strengthen her weak claw and hang on.

Then came the day I decided to wean Polly from relying on the tape. I explained to Chad that this was not going to be easy for her. When she tumbled off the first time, Chad looked at me and said, "Let's give her another chance." He tapped gently on her head, trying in his own way to give encouragement. This was a natural segue to talking about his problems and how he also needed to be determined and not give up. Like Polly, he had a second chance to mend himself.

After only a few months, Polly was perching successfully, and I called the veterinarian to tell her Polly was ready for adoption. When Chad heard this, he asked immediately if he could have her. He ran out of the room and called, "Mom, can we adopt Polly?" I knew Chad had genuine affection for Polly and had worked hard in helping her. I also knew Polly could help Chad, could be his inspiration. So with all of us in agreement, Chad officially adopted Polly. On the day he was to take her home his joy was infectious. But as a precaution, I had structured a transitional period for the two of them. Each day Chad was to call in a report. It worked out well. Polly filled a looming void in Chad's life, so it was a mutually beneficial relationship, and the effects spilled beyond the home. The kids on his block were impressed with his new friend and his knowledge and confidence in discussing her.

As Chad's therapy continued, he'd bring Polly into the office every three or four weeks to say a quick hello and, I suspect, for a grooming, as I always offered to trim Polly's wing feathers and nails. But I didn't really mind. I'd also grown fond of Polly and enjoyed seeing her.

Chad's progress increased, and over the next several months he blossomed. His school work improved, and he had learned how to handle the bullies at school without resorting to physical or verbal attacks, which in the past had only encouraged his tormenters. Without the necessary fuel the bullies delighted in, the attacks eventually stopped, and Chad discovered he could have positive interactions with his classmates. Through Polly, Chad learned that imperfection is okay, that it is all right to have flaws. However, we must accept that we have them and not allow those flaws to become obstacles for life's opportunities.

Over the course of the last four years I have interviewed folks from all over the world to learn about the healing power of the human-animal connection. I've discovered, like many others, that mending physically, emotionally, and spiritually are all important components to making a whole person again. One of the most heart-wrenching accounts I have heard is the unique relationship between an injured duck and an eight-year-old boy named John.

According to the therapist, the boy experienced tremendous trauma as a toddler. At the age of three, John and his two baby sisters (ages one and two) had been submerged into a bath filled with scalding water. The children screamed, but their mother did not pull them out. She reported thinking that they were just being stubborn about bathing.

All the children suffered third-degree burns over most of their bodies. John's youngest sister died immediately in the bath, and the other sister died one month later in the hospital. As for John, he suffered third-degree burns on his buttocks, legs, feet, and back. His mother was arrested and charged with murder, but the charges were eventually reduced to extreme and gross neglect.

John was hospitalized in the burn unit for quite a while. He underwent major skin graft surgeries. To complicate the matter, John was deaf since birth and the staff had a hard time communicating with him. Once released from the hospital, John was placed, unsuccessfully, in several foster homes. Because of his disruptive behavior he was eventually placed in a children's shelter, where he began to form meaningful relationships with the staff and a few other children.

But John's battle was not over. When he was six years old, he needed to have surgery once again to help with his healing because he was outgrowing the skin from the first grafts. The process was extremely traumatic for him because he didn't comprehend all that was happening to him and because he was removed from a place where he felt safe and secure. As a consequence of this trauma and the lack of stability in his life, he demonstrated significant evidence of depression and anger clearly related to his abusive history. John also showed distrust for many who cared for him, questioning their authority with disdain. His inability to communicate made matters worse, and John appeared to have difficulties distinguishing reality from fantasy. He was in need of productive therapy, and that is where the Forget Me Not Farm came into play.

He began attending the Humane Society's Forget Me Not Farm program on a weekly basis. Founded in 1992 at the Humane Society of Sonoma County, the site was established to teach children empathy and compassion through their interactions with animals and gardening. The program was designed to help abused children by immersing them in a nurturing environment where they could witness firsthand the miracles of plant growth, where animals could become their loving companions, and where they would meet and interact with adults who could be trustworthy mentors.

Initially he was frightened by the various animals, even kittens and puppies. Over the course of several weeks, however, John slowly grew attached to the baby animals. It was evident that he knew how to handle the young ones, perhaps because of his nurturing role with his deceased sisters. But for several months John continued to be frightened of the larger animals. Eventually he began to develop trust in one horse and allowed himself a ride. John was clearly exhilarated by his own ability to overcome this fear, as evidenced by his laughing and relating his experience to others. John also became more social, approaching the volunteers at Forget Me Not to tell them stories about himself and his experiences with the animals. However, his greatest conquest at the Farm was his relationship with an injured duck.

According to Carol Rathmann, the program director of the farm, John first discovered the duck accidentally on a rainy day when he went inside to use the bathroom. Once inside the building, John found the injured duck and appeared very curious about its well-being. He had many questions about why the duck was there, and through his interpreter, Carol tried to answer them all. Carol explained to John that the duck was put into the tub several times a week for exercise to help with a badly injured leg.

Over the next couple of months, the little duck was the highlight of John's visits to the farm. He would always run over to see how he was recovering. To get him more involved in the therapy, he was allowed to fill the tub and help put the duck into the water. Without apparent realization, John filled the tub with hot water. I'm sure his own experience with bathing was playing a part in his treatment of the duck. Carol spent many afternoons explaining to John that ducks normally swam outside in cold water, and he needed to pour cooler water into the tub. For several weeks he continued to try to make the water warmer. It took a while, but eventually he respected that the water needed to be cold.

As John began to understand how the water was helping the duck move around and exercise his bad leg, he tried several ways to encourage the duck to swim. One day when he was snacking on Goldfish crackers, John looked towards the duck and asked if he could give her one. Once he got the okay, he stretched his arm out to the waiting duck. To his delight the duck anxiously took as many crackers as John offered. He quickly discovered that the duck would swim towards him to get the crackers. His kindness and gentle response to the duck helped it get stronger, which in turn gave John more confidence. The duck eventually got well and began to swim more on his own, and John began to learn that he could trust others without harm to himself. In honor of John's technique, the Farm named the duck Crackers.

When the weather warmed up an outdoor swimming pool was created for Crackers. For his contribution, John was allowed to release Crackers into his new swimming area. As soon as Crackers hit the water he dived under, flapped his wings, tossed water all around, and did all of the normal duck behaviors. John was delighted and began smiling and laughing at Cracker's antics. John quickly reached in his pocket and shared a few more Goldfish crackers. The crackers were the treat that healed both of their broken souls. Crackers was now free to swim without impairments, and John's symbolic release of Crackers into the water perhaps helped him cleanse his soul of past trauma.

Getting a New Leash on Life—It Really Works!

Shoemakers resole shoes, mechanics fine-tune cars, and gardeners restore lawns. Each of these honored professions, like mental health professionals, helps rebuild and give new life to what once was disregarded and thought of as beyond repair. Some of us are lucky enough in life to get a second chance, a new beginning. In golf we would call this a Mulligan, or a re-do. Wouldn't it be great if we were afforded a new chance every time things didn't work out as expected? For many, second chances are plentiful, while for others they are not. Sometimes life's misfortunes can alter our future. The final part of this chapter will focus on the lucky folks who not only got a second chance, but also took advantage of it. Some don't even realize they are getting a second chance until a remarkable change occurs.

When I first met Puppy, she needed a second chance in life. If I had been too busy, too self-absorbed, or willing to let someone else do it, my life would have never been the same, and Puppy's would have remained shadowed by her abuse and neglect. But I believe in the human spirit and our ability to adapt and change. I have also gained an appreciation of what it takes to close a wound and help it to heal. All of us are the authors of our own stories, and hopefully we can pen endings that have healthy outcomes. There is really no such thing as coincidence: Puppy and I were fated to meet; I was meant to adopt and fall in love with her. Our love was meant to be.

Sometimes change happens through hard work and determination. Sometimes change occurs when we help others. While supporting others (or causes we care about) we begin to see more purpose and value in our lives, helping others while helping ourselves. This prescription for better physical and mental health has been known and used for centuries. When we pair the needy with those who can help, magic can occur, especially when direct action is taken. Here are a few examples.

Juan and Velma

In January 1999, Project Second Chance was developed at the Youth Diagnostic and Development Center (YDDC) in Albuquerque, New Mexico under the direction of Tamara Ward. Their goal is to help juveniles learn to explore their emotional health through interaction with animals. The YDDC is one of several juvenile correctional facilities throughout New Mexico which serves boys and girls (ages 12–21). Most of the youth are committed to the Center for one or two years; others remain until the age of twenty-one.

Project Second Chance operates seven times a year and is designed to last three weeks. The goal of the project is for selected adolescents to help a small group of dogs refine their behaviors so they can be adopted. During each session four shelter dogs are brought to the Center by the Humane Association. The dogs are boarded there for the three-week period. Once the animals arrive, each dog is paired with a resident, who becomes a mentor and teacher, responsible for the day-to-day care of the animal. The care includes maintaining the kennel, feeding, walking, and training his/her chosen dog.

Each mentor receives lessons in basic dog training (from the staff of the Project), and the emphasis is on positive reinforcement rather than aggression and negative punishment. Acknowledging the dog's past and becoming more empathetic are variables that are critical to the success of the project. At the completion of the program each mentor is asked to write a letter to a prospective adoptive family, sharing why he believes the dog deserves a second chance. The process of writing the letter helps bring closure and encourages the mentors to think about their role in the relationship and the impact it has had on their own life. Let's meet Juan, one the project's graduates, and his dog.

———

Velma, a tiny terrier cross-breed, is two years of age when she arrives at the YDDC. She looks terrified. She's panting hard and has her tail between her legs. Once escorted into the kennel, she walks cautiously to the corner, isolating herself from the pack. She looks pathetic, hopeless, and helpless, beaten into a role of fear and submission. Velma has had a harsh beginning to her life. She's been removed from her home because of abuse and neglect. Her long hair is completely matted to her small body. Velma has been conditioned to fear humans, and this needs to change if she has any hope of being adopted. Velma needs a second chance. She needs a mentor who can gain her trust and show her that she is loveable and that not all humans are to be distrusted.

When the four trainers arrived at the kennel to select their dogs, Velma was the third to be shown. Although she was shaking with fear, Juan was drawn to her and made his choice. The next day he found Velma again sitting alone in the corner. The staff coached Juan to enter and sit in the middle of the floor. He glanced shyly at Velma and in a soft voice called, "It'll be all right, girl, it's all right. Come to me. Come on girl, come." But Velma sat as if frozen in place and trembled. Juan repeated his words but got no response. In the past Juan would have lashed out; this is his history. He's been the abuser in past relationships, but he knew not to do this to her. At the same time, Juan didn't know what to do; he had no experience to call on. With encouragement Juan realized, as with himself, that Velma was responsible for her behavior, not his lack of skill.

While the other students made progress, Juan spent most of his time trying to gain Velma's trust, and each day did bring progress. But not until two weeks into the program did Velma feel comfortable enough with Juan to follow him and allow him to hold her. They were getting closer to their goal, but time was not on their side. Juan even took extra time to work with Velma. However, at the end of the three weeks, Velma was still not ready for adoption and was sent to a transitional foster home.

Juan's experience had been so moving that he asked for another opportunity. Because he showed patience, diligence, and kindness toward Velma, the Center, in an unprecedented move, granted Juan another chance. This time his dog was named Rascal. About the same size as Velma, she was very happy and liked humans. Her background is one of survivor rather than victim, and Juan found her much more open to training. Juan successfully trained Rascal and she left the program to start a new life with a loving family.

When asked about his short time with Velma and Rascal, Juan spent more time focusing on Velma. Perhaps he was closer with Velma because she was so needy and he saw connections between himself and her—the abuser and the abused. He also saw within Velma those he had hurt in the past. But now the abuser understands what the victim experiences.

Gazing at the ceiling when asked about Velma and getting a second chance, he said, "You know, I really spent time thinking about what I needed to give a dog like Velma so she could become more secure.

Probably the most important ingredient that I had to show her was that my intentions were friendly. I had to show her that I would not harm her like those people in her past. I also had to help her realize that she could trust me because I would treat her in a calm, gentle and loving manner."

He continued, "I think my experience with Velma will help me relate with other dogs and kids. I used to smack dogs and kids on their butts to get them to do what I wanted them to do. But after being around Velma I now know that I shouldn't do that anymore. I cannot use violence. Violence may get people to listen to me, but they won't trust me or want to be around me."

In a subsequent conversation Juan shared new insights. Perhaps he had displaced these feelings over the years, but working with Velma helped them surface.

You know, there are some other similarities between the Velma and myself that I have never shared. Although she was a victim and I was an abuser, it seemed that one thing we had in common was that we had both been rejected. Once I began to understand that, it became clear to me that the sense of rejection we both once felt was the element that connected our souls. I tried to do things for her that I knew would help me. Using sensitivity was not something that I usually practiced. In the past it was much easier for me to blow up and be hurtful. Working with Velma took a lot of patience, but I didn't give up on her. My reward was that in time she began to trust me more.

I wish I could have had more time with her, but I do understand that more time would have made it very difficult for us to separate. So perhaps it was better that she moved into the foster home. Although I still feel her loss, it is now a good feeling. I now know what it might feel like to be a dad, to teach a child you need to be gentler rather than always using a hard hand.

There are so many things I would like to talk about in looking back at my moments with Velma. When I was working with her, not the training part, but the bonding parts were the most memorable moments I look back at. I remember sitting on the grass in her kennel and talking to her, spending time and petting her head. She looked at me like I was the man in her world. Over the time when we just began to bond it seemed like she knew I wanted to be her friend. It's amazing that this shy, timid and fearful dog learned from me. I also should be grateful to her. She opened my eyes to the gift of kindness. It took courage for her to try to trust people. It took seeing and feeling her fear for me to realize the mistakes of my past and that I could change too!"

Green Chimneys: Nancy

"Mom, I'm going to my room to do homework. Keep an eye on Blizzard for me, okay?" Nancy's mom, Eva, replies, "Sure, I'll be right here." Blizzard's an eighteen-month-old golden retriever that Nancy has been training for East Coast Assistance Dogs (ECAD). On the weekends Blizzard comes home with Nancy. This evening Blizzard continues lying on her rug as Nancy leaves the room. When Eva least expects it, Blizzard jumps onto the couch, snuggling next to her. Eva's first reaction is to laugh and tell the dog to get down, but she immediately remembers Nancy's warning not to laugh when giving Blizzard commands. Nancy takes training seriously and has tried to stress the importance of consistent training to her family. She has even gone so far as to post a list of commands on the fridge. But as on many other occasions, Eva can't remember the correct one. Is it "down" or "off"? She runs towards the kitchen to look. Or, she thinks, I can just call Nancy for help. Then she laughs to herself and thinks, "Wow! Things have sure changed in this house."

When Nancy was fourteen years old, she began attending Green Chimney's therapeutic day program. The Southern Westchester County School District had referred Nancy to the program for a number of reasons. Diagnosed with a learning disability that was impacting her schoolwork, she also struggled with attention, organization, and poor social skills. Nancy was impulsive and could not recognize social boundaries. The defining factor in sending her to Green Chimneys was her hospitalization for self-abuse.

After a month or so of attending the day program, she returned to the hospital and was eventually discharged back into the school system. But while attending, she needed constant supervision to prevent fighting, other disruptive behavior, and continued self-abuse. The latter was cause enough to send her back to Green Chimneys.

112

In September 2002 she showed interest in participating in their training program for service dogs. Nancy recalls her reasons for asking about the program: "When I first started in the ECAD program two years ago, I knew something good could happen to change my future. I've loved animals since I was young. Whenever I saw programs on TV about working dogs helping people, I thought how great it would be to help dogs learn to do that."

Nancy's first dog was a chubby yellow Lab with very soft ears named Snow. The first time she met Snow she noticed a lack of spunk and personality. Snow looked depressed and was easily frustrated in training. "I grew frustrated with Snow, but I also thought she was like me. She wasn't able to show her frustration. Luckily, Dale was there to help me and encourage me not to give up or get mad at either Snow or myself. In the end, I learned as much from the training as Snow did."

At home, Eva saw the difference in Nancy. "She was always talking about training Snow. We could all see how much she loved it." Over the two years Nancy has continued to grow and learn. "Our family sees how her relationships with adults have changed. She has also had to learn to be consistent and patient."

Nancy now looks to the future, a future that will include animals. She has found a passion and a skill. Nancy closes her story with this statement:

> With the ECAD and the help of Dale I'm a better person and a great dog trainer. I never knew I could be so patient and motivated about something. Through the program, I started to behave better, to feel more confident, and to believe in miracles. Although it's hard sometimes to separate from the dogs I've trained, I only have to remind myself of the purpose—to provide loving, trustworthy partners for people in need. It makes me feel so good to know that I've helped someone.

Green Chimneys: Harvey

At the age of two years, Harvey was removed from his parents' custody and spent most of his developing years in the child welfare system of New York state. He spent time at various residential facilities and was bounced in and out of the foster care system. After being expelled from eight schools by the age of nine, Harvey was sent to Green Chimneys. He describes himself during this time as quiet, short tempered, and disruptive. Although he appeared tough on the outside, inside he yearned for closer relationships. He states, "I was very open to anyone who was accepting of me because I didn't have any parents." However, without any strong parental models to mold his behavior and relieve his anger, most relationships failed.

This was evident to the staff at Green Chimneys. He refused to talk to anyone, especially the staff and therapists. The residence did, however, have one attraction for Harvey: the animals. He soon realized that the only way to gain access to these animals was by interacting with the staff, to ask for help and permission. "That started a kind of chain reaction. The more I communicated with the staff, the more time I could spend with the animals. Although the therapists did help me, I got more comfort from the interaction with the animals, and, on some level, I felt we had something in common."

Although drawn to all of the wildlife there, Harvey was most attracted to the horses. His first experience was with a horse named Laddie. "When I first saw Laddie my initial reaction was, 'This horse is going to kick my butt.' I was afraid it would trample my feet. The relationship with a horse is slow to establish at first; you need to learn how to trust it and let the horse learn to trust you. Never in my life did I think I'd ever care for a horse, much less learn to ride one."

Harvey says he was first attracted to Laddie because her golden color stood out from the other horses'. He soon found out, though, that horses sense quickly if you're afraid. As his relationship with Laddie blossomed he learned new activities and how to control his fear. He states, "It was important to recognize that animals have feelings and that they were at Green Chimneys for the same reason I was, to get better."

Harvey took advantage of every animal program offered at the facility. One of his favorites was the Farmer on the Move program, in which the animals of Green Chimneys traveled to different places to show and teach others. He says he felt a sense of pride in being able to give other kids the same type of experience he had, especially those living in large cities. Harvey feels he grew emotionally from this program and that his confidence increased because he could teach others. "I had to take what I learned and apply it to others. I had to practice how to conduct myself in public."

From this experience Harvey now thinks about a positive future: "I'm more accepting of others." Today, Harvey is a college student majoring in communications with a minor in business. His social life is full of friends, and his interests range from participating on the wrestling team to playing chess. Although he's no longer a resident at Green Chimneys, he remains an active member of the community. Recently, he traveled to Arizona as a spokesperson, where he now works during the summer.

Harvey is aware of his past and is not shy about sharing his experience with others so that they may learn from it. Recently, he reunited with his parents and plans on staying in contact with them because he "values all relationships."

Derek and Noah

It was a warm summer evening when our paths crossed again. It was a night for celebration. Derek is now eighteen and has come home as a high school graduate. His battle to reach this milestone was an arduous journey, one with several detours. I see that Derek has changed physically since I last saw him; he has plugs in his ears and looks much more like a young man. He has a pack of cigarettes in his hands but decides to return them to his car. "I don't think you would appreciate these," he chuckles. "Things have really changed for me, mostly for the better. I now realize I don't have to have a front; I can just be me. I have worked very hard to make some life changes, and I just want to be happy."

Derek and I haven't seen each other for close to two years, but we have stayed in touch. In fact, it was Derek who inspired the name for PJ (Puppy Junior). Derek and I met when he was seven. His mother called me because he was struggling at a small private school. The staff viewed his behavior as deliberately unruly and disrespectful. He was also having difficulty keeping up with his classmates. He was diagnosed later that year as having Tourette's syndrome, which along with the associated vocal and motor tics, also consists of an array of behavioral challenges. Derek had trouble feeling good about himself, and to counter these challenges, he would show off, often at inappropriate times.

When I first met Derek, he was a very angry boy, and, frankly, it was easy to dislike him. He would often act boisterously, loud and off-color, both intentionally and unintentionally. But I saw beneath his surface behavior to a boy who needed help. He needed to like who he was so that others could see and hear beyond the Tourette's.

Over the years, I became one of his biggest advocates, arguing with school officials about his right to an appropriate education and working with his family to overcome their discouragement. Sometimes I was more successful than others. Derek was a challenge, and although we made progress, there were also setbacks, especially when he got into his teen years. They were the most turbulent for him, as with many of us, but his behavior eventually led to his placement at the Colorado Boy's Ranch, a therapeutic living community for young men. His departure was hard for me, but I knew a more consistent and structured environment was best for him.

At sixteen, Derek resented going to the ranch, but on some level he knew that he needed this experience to change his unhealthy lifestyle. When we reminisced that evening he told me about his anger. He said his first night was awful. He felt his parents had abandoned him and he was afraid. It took Derek some time to adjust to Colorado. At first he did not open up to the staff or residents. Once again, many of those around him took a dislike to his attitude and behavior and, therefore, to the boy.

Eventually Derek entered the Ranch's dog training program, which is longer (ten weeks) but similar to the one Juan participated in. The program is held daily for an hour and a half, and the emphasis is on learning to build relationships as well as readying dogs for adoption.

Noah wasn't Derek's first choice, but most of the dogs had already been chosen. Noah didn't make a good first impression. His hair was shaggy and filled with knots. Derek explains, "When I saw him for the first time it was just one of those things. You know. You look at something and go 'Ugh.' I just wanted to walk away, walk past the kennel. I couldn't stand the thought of touching him. But then I decided I might as well give it a try, so I walked into his kennel. When I looked at his face and into those eyes—well, it was love at first sight." As Derek told me more about Noah, I began to understand. He was a white poodle with a red scar around his muzzle caused when the previous owner shut his mouth with rubber bands so he wouldn't bark. Like Velma, Noah was wary of humans, but the more Derek worked with him, the more the dog warmed up to him.

The first day, Derek entered the kennel and just sat on the ground. To his surprise, Noah wandered towards him. "When he came up to me and sat on my lap, it was one of the most moving experiences in my life. I knew he liked me, and maybe for the first time I began to realize that I was a worthwhile person. I even started crying, remembering things back home. From that day forward I realized that although I was to be his savior, in reality he was also going to be mine. He made me realize that I had value and I needed to change my life. I really wonder now just who picked who for this project."

Derek's progress can be seen in his approach to Noah. Because the dog was easily frightened and distracted, Derek decided to work with him in a quieter, more secluded place. As the bond between them grew, he spent more time working and playing with Noah. He even taught him tricks. His two favorite tricks were teaching him to play dead and running through a six-foot tunnel. To play dead he would tap the ground and Noah would fall down and stay still. He used a clicker to signal Noah that he had done what he was supposed to and then followed this with a reward. "He's like me. When I wash cars, I love when people tell me I did a great job. It lets you know you are appreciated."

As the program came to a close, Derek knew it would be hard to say goodbye to Noah. He had successfully trained Noah, but this success was bittersweet. Only after the graduation ceremony did the parting really sink in—Noah was gone from his life. His one consolation had been that he'd had a part in picking Noah's new family, and although saddened by his loss, Derek was comfortable with his choice and knew Noah would be happy.

After a few weeks Derek visited Noah at his new home. He was ambivalent about the meeting but was excited to see his pal and see how he was doing. Derek started calling Noah's name before he even stepped into the house and Noah immediately knew who it was. Derek told me, "Noah's little tail would not stop wagging. As soon as I sat down, he jumped in my lap and licked my face. It really touched my heart. He recognized me and knew who I was." They visited for a while, but Derek was careful not to disturb Noah's new routine at the house. He knew he'd have to leave soon and didn't want Noah upset. Derek still keeps in contact with Noah's family and is planning a trip to Colorado in the near future.

Later that evening Derek confided to me, "The thing I'll miss the most about Noah is his love and compassion for me. I felt abandoned when I went to Colorado and Noah had been abandoned as well. We have this great connection, a great relationship."

In many ways it was good for Derek to see Noah happy. It gave him closure and allowed him to acknowledge that he had gone a good job. We drank a few more Cokes that evening and talked about all the changes that had occurred in his life. Derek was still comfortable with talking to me. He said, "You always knew it was easier for me to express myself with the animals than people. Puppy always loved me for who I was. I didn't have to show off for her." I agreed but reflected, "Puppy was a great influence, but Noah was the saving grace." As I bid Derek goodbye, I thought about the boy and the dog, about two lost souls that needed mending and a second chance.

Bark Insight

We know everyone deserves a second chance, a re-do in life. Things may not always work out the way we want them to the first time around, but that doesn't mean we have to give up! We usually have two choices. One choice leaves us feeling empty and unfulfilled, while the other alternative leaves us filled with hope. That sense of hope allows us to realize a new beginning and a new tomorrow. I have to tell you that taking chances and opening yourself up can be scary when you first try, but that shouldn't get in your way.

When I sit back and think about it, I always wonder where I would have been if life hadn't given me a second go. For that matter, where would I have been if I hadn't opened up and taken a chance? I hated myself and didn't feel worthwhile. I was afraid of touch and believed that no one could be trusted. Over time, I found someone that did give me a chance. He showed me that he wouldn't hurt me and that life could be fair, but I had to open up and let the goodness come to me. My life has never been the same. I feel that what I learned made a difference to others.

Everyone needs to realize that life is worthwhile. In a time when things don't work out, my suggestion is to realize that it is okay to try again. Failure is an event. We must not personalize our failures and identify with them. It is okay to make mistakes, especially when we try to learn from them. Second chances are gifts from heaven. We need to be willing to give them to those in need and to accept them if we are in need.

Throughout this chapter you read about dogs and birds, boys and girls, who learned from their new chances and changed their own lives. I was touched when I heard the stories. Rather than wallowing in self-pity, we need to take chances and move forward. My advice to you is to realize that you are only on the merry-go-round of life once, so you'd better make the best of it. I should know because the last ten years of my life were the best! I finally realized that I was a lovable and capable creature. Learn from me. A soul is always worth mending. A soul is always worth saving. I should know—I was saved. Since then my mission was to help people see their light and their life possibilities. I am grateful for my second chance. By the way, my name is Puppy.

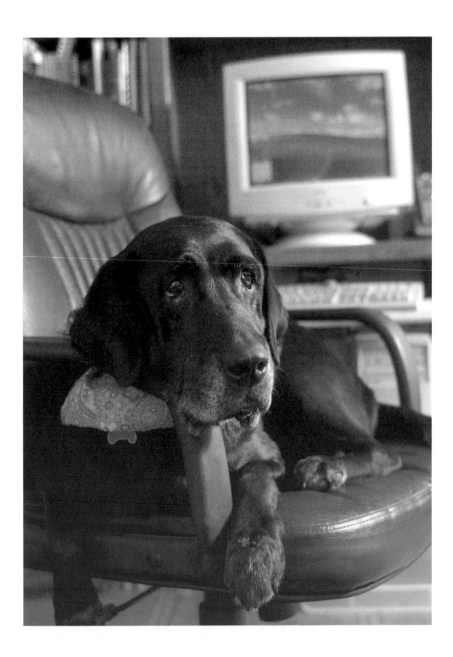

Writing from the Hart

Becoming a Cyrano de Bergerac

Now it's my turn to give you the pep talk, to give you the confidence to leave with a positive attitude and a healthy mind-set. I am so proud of you! I hope you'll jump right into your studies and get the most out of your experience. Life is all about opening and closing doors. This is your chance to get a new start and open a few doors!

Well, have a safe trip. Remember to take care of yourself, eat, exercise and have fun. It is important to have balance. I'll be waiting to hear from my pal. I know how hard it is to leave but I know I will see you soon. Life is like a boomerang. Things always come back. I know when I see you again, you might be a little older and wiser, but you still will be my sweet little boy. Follow your dreams and make things happen.

I love you my little, big boy. Be safe and I will be waiting to rock with you in your truck and cuddle in your bed when our paths cross again. I love you!!!!

With all my heart,

> *Love,*
>
> *Hart*

———

It seems like only yesterday that I began writing letters to my sons in the guise of one of our dogs. I thought it was a great idea. What could be more powerful than receiving a note from one of our four-legged family members? Of course, the boys knew it was me, and I suppose, if I'm perfectly honest, writing the notes was more for me than them because this method made it easier for me to express my feelings. Sometimes the notes were meant to be amusing, while other times they were intended to motivate and console. Although both boys have been the recipients of numerous letters, it was the writings from Hart to Corey that influenced me to apply this strategy as part of my therapy practice. This tradition has continued ever since, and I presently write letters weekly to many of my clients to inspire them to work hard and persevere. Receiving a card from Dr. Fine might be nice, but getting a personal letter from their beloved therapy dog has more meaning.

Over the years I have written notes to let children know how much they were appreciated; to encourage children to work harder at school, and to try to modify their behavior with family. Amusing notes have been sent to youngsters when celebrating a special event in their lives such as a birthday, prom, or sporting event. Letters have also been written to congratulate not only clients, but also their parents, and my family and friends, for special occasions such as graduating from school, getting married, joining the armed services and having a child.

Ultimately, the letters have helped me cultivate a unique dimension to my therapeutic relationships with my clients. It has allowed me to communicate not only as an adult authority figure, but also as a friend. My letters have met with success. Who hasn't imagined what a beloved pet would say if it could talk? Writing under a pseudonym is a time-honored tradition, and speaking through my dogs works on a couple of levels, just as it did for Cyrano de Bergerac.

For those of you only familiar with Edmond Rostandt's play or one of the film adaptations, Cyrano de Bergerac is not a fictional character. He was a charming soldier with the tremendous gift of writing and charm. However, although he was blessed with these gifts, he lacked self-confidence because of his physical appearance. Although it might be exaggerated in the play and films, he did have a large nose. As the story goes, Cyrano provides a handsome fellow soldier, Christian, the words with which to woo Roxanne, the beautiful woman they both are in love with. Cyrano's eloquence in writing the letters, signed by Christian, is successful in winning Roxanne's love and affection. Without going into too many details about the actual play, after many years, and the death of Christian, Roxanne and Cyrano meet. She then realizes he was the author of the letters and that it is he, Cyrano, whom she loves.

Using a pseudonym allows a certain freedom, especially if we are shy. But it is also just plain fun. Like my sons, my patients know I write the notes but they enjoy the fantasy, and, as I did when writing to my boys, I often feel freer to address their frustration as well as their joy. I find the correspondence helpful and invigorating and hope after reading this sampling you do as well.

Letters to My Sons
College

Dear Corey:

Having time is a treasure we all have to cherish. In our case, limited time is the enemy. We never have enough of it, and the next few days will not be an exception. I hate to say goodbyes. It was hard enough six years ago when I was a little girl and you were bringing me to the kennel for the last time. I thought I would never see you again, but with fortune (not for Guide Dogs) our lives crossed again. It has been fun growing up with "my little boy," who has become my best human friend.

The last time I wrote you a long letter, you were the boy I would never forget. You had become my soul mate, the human that showed me beauty in life. You helped me learn right from wrong, got me out of jams when I was in them, but most of all you played with me and gave me lots of loving. Even as you have aged, you still made time for me. I feel so special, especially when we hang out! I have been a pretty lucky girl to have been able to steal your heart for such a long time.

Goodbyes are so hard, especially for me! Maybe we shouldn't look at this as a goodbye, but a chance for you to fly on your own. When I was young and it was my time to leave, you hugged me and told me that you gave me what I needed so I could handle it. With love, kindness and lots of attention, you gave me the confidence I needed, so that when I left, I wasn't afraid.

Now it's my turn to give you the pep talk, to give you the confidence to leave with a positive attitude and a healthy mind-set. I am so proud of you! I hope you'll jump right into your studies and get the most out of your experience. Life is all about opening and closing doors. This is your chance to get a new start and open a few doors!

Well, have a safe trip. Remember to take care of yourself, eat, exercise and have fun. It is important to have balance. I'll be waiting to hear from my pal. I know how hard it is to leave but I know I will see you soon. Life is like a boomerang. Things always come back. I know when I see you again, you might be a little older and wiser, but you still will be my sweet little boy. Follow your dreams and make things happen.

I love you my little, big boy. Be safe and I will be waiting to rock with you in your truck and cuddle in your bed when our paths cross again. I love you!!!!

With all my heart,

Love;

Hart

Not Giving Up

My dear Corey:

What do you think? Do you like my new cards? Shrimp and I look great! We may be getting older, but we are good looking!

I've enjoyed having you home on your break from school. You make me feel so special. I hope I still make you feel great too.

Barks (or you would say words) do not describe how I love you. I have watched you grow up to become a beautiful young man. I know that times can get tough when you get older, but you have to believe in the good. Never let things get you down. You are too good for that! People (and dogs too) are lucky to have you in their lives.

Well, I still have you for a more days before you need to leave again. Give me lots and lots of attention. I really want it, especially when we go for the drives. I love sticking my head out of the truck window. Remember one thing: you are my special human—my true first and best friend.

I love you.

Hart

Making Decisions

Dear Sean:

Decisions, decisions, why are they so hard to make? Even more, why do we begin to doubt ourselves once we make a choice? Listen, my big 2-legged brother; life is filled with so

many mysteries. Remember "we always don't know what we are going to get."

You know me, Miss Chicken Little, always afraid of new things, but I am starting to learn that if you want something new in life, you have to take chances. Chances are not all that bad. They are a little scary at first, but in most cases they do work out. When you select a certain pathway, you will never really know what the other options would have brought you.

But the treasures of life shouldn't be just tinsel and tin. You have to feel good about your life experiences. I wanted to write to lend you a supportive paw. You know that we are all here to support you. Things worth having sometimes have a cost. Don't worry about how it will be paid for. We will all lend a hand. The gang will give up some of our treats and bones to chip in. In most cases things have a way of working themselves out. But you have to give them a chance.

Take the time over the next several months and celebrate what you accomplished. Relax and smell the roses. Come by and take us for a few walks. We'll help you relax and keep your mind healthy.

We love you bunches,

PJ and Hart

A Letter from My Son

The tradition of writing letters to my sons continues. Although they are now adults, they continue to be amused when they receive a note from one of our beloved family dogs. But have also they learned to read between the lines. Some of the notes are filled with amusing and loving messages while others are more thought-provoking and related to issues that they are dealing with. Of course, they saw through this device quickly, but looked forward to them, much as they did with the tooth fairy. The notes encourage my sons to think and smile, but most importantly, the messages let them know I care and I am thinking about them.

The boys have found this outlet a valuable alternative for the more traditional forms of conversations and communication. They have found this approach so useful that they have elected periodically to write notes to me. The notes, signed by one of the dogs, help them express their feelings and possible concerns. Just as with the boys, reading the notes often makes me smile and reflect upon what was written.

The following letter is one simple example. Over the years, I have battled with my weight. I work out and exercise diligently, but I periodically lose direction and munch (my wife would possibly use an alternative term). I have at times felt like a family project: "prevent Dad from snacking." I realize that in most cases, the kids and my wife have my best interest in mind. Nevertheless, I periodically get my feelings hurt or get annoyed. The following note was received after one of those bouts. It was written by my older son, who seemed to be bothered after our interaction. He didn't want to hurt my feelings, but rather help guide me to stay the course. After reading this note, I took to heart what he was saying. Perhaps it was because it was disguised as my dear little PJ. Here is the note:

Dear Daddy,

Sean talked to me earlier and told me that he may have upset you. He asked me to write this letter to you because like everyone knows, I am your little princess. I know it is hard for you sometimes because you love food, just like I love my cookies. I COULD EAT ALL DAY LONG, but I know in the end that it would not be good for me because I could get sick and may go to the bathroom all over the house. I know Mom would get really mad at me. When the family bugs you a little bit about your eating habits, they are not doing it to make fun of you or give you a hard time, but they are doing it because they love you and care about you so much. It is almost like when I was scared about going to the vet and spent fifteen meetings avoiding going into the office (I even tried to take off and run, but didn't get too far), Mom got really annoyed with me. After thinking about the day when I got home that evening, I realized that she was not yelling at me because she was mad. She acted harshly because she cared about my safety. I know it is hard when you get others' disapproval (believe me, I KNOW THAT), but we should listen to what others say. They are words and often aren't intended to hurt.

I just wanted to let you know that I am here for you and love you so much. I also want to make sure that you know that the whole family loves you, even if they sometimes give you a tough time about food. You know one thing for sure, I love you bunches!!

Love,
Your Princess

PJ

This note touched me deeply. My hurt feelings had already disappeared, but receiving this letter reaffirmed my love for the boys. They not only care but are concerned. Here is my brief reply, a copy of an e-mail sent to my older son.

Hey PJ,

Thanks for the note. You are really my star. Sometimes emotions are good because they let people know how you feel. It is hard for me, as it is for you, to control the urges. Even when I give it the best effort, it sometimes is a battle. I know you understand this, because I try to exercise you a lot. I guess we can only do the best we can! I want to let you know how much I love getting these letters from you. They help me put things into perspective, especially when things are tough. Always know that you have a very special place in my heart, especially because I know you care!

Love you, Princess—or should I say, Prince.

Dad

Being a Pen Pal

It was the middle of September (several years ago) when Lindsey's mother initially contacted me. She was worried about her daughter, who would often be overheard saying such things as, "I hate myself," "I'm so ugly," and "No one likes me." During the summer vacation, Lindsey was registered in a day camp. For weeks she came home unhappy, even depressed. One day, Lindsey told her mother that the other campers were picking on her and she flatly refused to go back. She spent the rest of the summer at home, alone except for family.

When she started school that fall, the teasing didn't stop, and it was evident that Lindsey wasn't equipped to cope. A few of the boys were making fun of her weight, which devastated her. She'd sulk for days after an incident, and this had ramifications on her home and school life. Her mother was at a loss, unable to help Lindsey with her problems, so I agreed to work with Lindsey.

At our first meeting I observed she was pulling inward. She put on a show of having a bubbly personality, but she avoided making eye contact and spoke little. Along with a weight problem, Lindsey had a pronounced lisp, of which she was also self-conscious. Confirmation of her struggle came when I asked her to draw a picture of herself at school. She drew herself larger than any of her classmates, but what was significant was that she drew herself as separated from her classmates. Her low self-esteem and sense of isolation were going to be the main focus of her therapy.

After a few weeks, our afternoon sessions fell into a routine: I would greet Lindsey and her mom in the waiting room, sometimes by myself and sometimes with PJ and Hart. Lindsey's first question coming in the door was always: "Are the dogs here?" If they were, joyous pandemonium ensued as Lindsey knelt on the floor to embrace PJ. The more patient and low-keyed Hart waited for her turn quietly. If the dogs weren't there, Lindsey would frown slightly, disappointed at not receiving her customary welcome, but, surprisingly, she didn't sulk. She knew that the dogs would come sometime during her session, and that awareness was enough for her.

Although she loved both dogs, she identified most closely with PJ. I believe this was because PJ, who was still a relatively young dog—less than two years old—often got into minor trouble with her small acts of "puppy" mischief. Lindsey found this both amusing and reassuring. Sometimes when Lindsey and I entered the back office for our session, we found paper from my trashcan strewn around the floor. PJ, looking slightly guilty, would hang back, waiting to see how I reacted. After a mild exclamation, like "Uh-oh," I would kneel on the floor, picking up the paper and putting it back in the trashcan. PJ would then come over to me and lick my face as I finished cleaning up. "Thank you, PJ," I'd say as Lindsey giggled. The way that I responded to PJ's mistakes intrigued Lindsey. I could tell that she was charmed by the unconditional love and trust that PJ and I shared.

Lindsey's relationship with PJ was an important aspect of her therapy and was further cemented when the two became pen pals. Since Lindsey had trouble expressing her feelings and needed practice writing legibly, we decided that Lindsey should write PJ a letter each week. This assignment was an unqualified success. Sometimes Lindsey wrote simple notes telling PJ about her day. At other times, she asked PJ for advice with problems she was facing. Here are a few examples of the notes.

Dear PJ and Hart,

I miss you a lot. You know what? I watch Animal Planet. At school older boys always say mean things to me. They say I can't do math. But I can. What should I do? I just got back from school so I need to finish my homework. Write back soon. Bye.

Love,
Lindsey

P.S. Dogs rule!

PJ's response:

Dear Lindsey,

When I was in school at my first obedience class, I was the youngest dog there. Lots of the older dogs and even their humans—who you think would know better—made fun of me. I wasn't very good at following all the commands. How could I "sit" when there were other dogs to play with? Why "stay" when the park was so full of such interesting smells? They thought I couldn't do the commands, but I really could!

I decided I wouldn't pay attention to the other dogs and their humans. That's when I really began to get the hang of the class. I didn't give up and I didn't let anyone bother me. I graduated. Dr. Fine has my diploma hanging on the wall at home. I am very proud of it.

If you just ignore the boys, then it won't matter if they say things. I know you can do it! Tell me how it goes.

Love,

PJ

Over time, Lindsey was encouraged to share the good things that happened in her life too.

Hi Lindsey,

How are you doing? Things are great here. Yesterday I got into a little trouble. I snuck into the cupboard and ate a half a box of dog cookies. They were great but today I have a tummy ache. Dr. Fine didn't even get mad at me, but he was worried I would get sick. Thank goodness I haven't (except for my tummy ache).

Hope you are doing well. Write soon and let me know what you have been up to. I really want to know how you are doing in school. Have you made any new friends? Say hi to your mom.

Your pal PJ

Lindsey's response:

Hey PJ,

I am doing great in math. The work has been pretty easy lately. How is your tummy feeling now? I hope you are feeling better. I have been so busy playing with my friends that I am never home. In school I am the helper in English class. I like helping the other kids. It makes me feel good. My mom is going to show me your website after we finish this email. I bet the website is going to be really, really cool. Say hi to Dr. Fine and Hart.

Love

Lindsey

One of the goals we worked on was overcoming negative thinking. I call these negative thoughts "whispering phantoms," and Lindsey had to learn to ignore them. Over the course of a year Lindsey probably wrote to PJ 25–30 times. She enjoyed being PJ's pen pal and would often just update her on how things were going. At times she would even write PJ to tell her about her work on therapeutic goals.

Dear PJ,

How are you doing? I'm doing great!!! I get to go to one of my friend's house in a little while. Did you know that I think you are the best dog in the world!! How many dogs write letters (ha-ha). Those phantoms don't bother me anymore! I feel much better because they aren't there anymore! I play softball much better now that they aren't there to bug me anymore! If I do hear those monsters I'll tell them DON"T BOTHER ME AND GO AWAY!!!! Then I just smile and forget about it!

Love,

Lindsey

PS— PJ you are the coolest of the coolest

Dear Lindsey:

I love mail.. Yeah, I got a few from you in the past few days. Keep on writing and don't forget: IGNORE THOSE ICHY PHANTOMS—THEY ARE REALLY MEAN. Thanks for calling me the coolest of the coolest. I will have to remember that when Shrimp and Hart try to boss me around.

YOUR PAL,

PJ

Lindsey is just one of the many children who made the dogs their confidants. Over the past five years, PJ has had several other pen pals.

Some just like to write to get a return note from her while others have more specific reasons. One girl began to write PJ to talk about her parents' divorce.

Dear Kimberly,

Thanks for the note. I love getting mail! Hope you have a great weekend. Today I had to take a bath. It felt good, but I hate the hair dryer. It makes a lot of noise. In your next letter to me, why don't you try to explain what divorce is to a girl like you? What is hard for you, and how can people make it better? As a dog, I never really lived with my real mom and dad. My human parents are great and I love being with them. I know it would be hard for me to not be able to see them a lot.

I am happy that you are visiting your dad more at your house. What do you like to do with him? I know he left when you were young, so you don't know all the things he likes. What would you want to tell him about you?

Maybe you could write to me and tell me what kind of family you would like to have. When you write to me, it will help me understand better. Well, I will see you soon.

PJ

Dear PJ,

I do not know what I really want in a family. All I can ever remember is living with my mother and sister. I love living with them, even if my sister bugs me. They are really nice! I think my family is great. Right now I like seeing my dad, but I really don't know him well. I like when he takes me on bike rides and just plays games with me, like card and board games. We also go to the park and play in the field. I still don't know what he likes a lot because I do not see him often. I see my dad about one day a week and that has only been for the last few months. I don't remember when he left because I was pretty small. Right now its fun when he is here. Sometimes he even gets us snacks. My dad buys us ice cream. He will give you cookies if you come over. I know you like cookies.

I will write you more later. I have to go and eat dinner.

Lindsey

The following letters are written to and from various children, and friends. I've grouped them into topics and events that happen to us all.

Friendship

Hey Girlfriend:

How was the weekend? I can't wait to see you and get filled in on the prom. I know you must have looked great! Did you get your hair and nails done? The blue gown sounds really pretty. What kind of corsage did your date get you?

Well, let's get to the main point. Was the food good? You know me, always thinking of those "cookies." I wish I could have gone. Sure the dancing and company would have been great, but the eating, well, I would have been in tenth heaven!

Hopefully you will have time this week to study for that big biology test you have on Thursday. If you need some help, you can come over to the office and I can watch you make some note cards and listen to you read out loud.

Have a great week and don't forget to fill me in on all the details when I see you next.

Your pal,

PJ

A letter from Sally, whom we discussed in the chapter "Do You Believe in Magic":

Dear Magic:

Thank you for letting me take you for a walk. I enjoy walking because you like me and lick me. Magic, you make me feel like a good girl because I am your eacher.

I like to visit you because May, Rachel and Mary come with me. They all make me laugh. I worried about PJ's foot when it got hurt. I was happy that you got a bandage on it.

I like when I get the chance to brush your hair. You are funny when you get your teeth brushed. I like it when I brush my teeth. I remember the time when I told PJ to sit when she was next to me. I was surprised when she jumped onto the couch right next to me. I laughed a lot. I laugh now when I think about that time. PJ was just listening to me.

When I met you, I was scared a little. I know you are nice, but I was scared. Now I know you are nice. I like you. I make you some pictures. I hope you like them.

    Love you.

Magic's response:

My dear friend Sally: My Teacher

I was so glad to receive your letter today. I am still a puppy, so I had PJ read it for me. She is now writing this note. I hope she is writing exactly what I say. You know PJ, she may be pulling a prank on me. Big sisters, they always want you to know who the boss is.

    *Well, I really loved the note and the picture you drew for me. I look pretty good in your drawing. I like that you drew us together taking a walk. I love going on walks with you, especially when you talk to me. You make me feel like the **bestest** dog in the world, when you tell me I am doing a good job! You know you are becoming a good teacher. So many people have tried to teach me things, but I really love how hard you are trying! I know when we first met you were a little nervous and afraid when we moved closer to you. I want you to always know that we are very gentle. Goldens are just balls of loving fur.*

    Have you noticed when you brush my fur how I almost fall asleep? I love when you do that. You brush so gently, just the way I like it. I know how careful you are trying to be, so that is why I stay so still. Boy, that is hard for me to do. Sally, let me ask you a question. What's with wanting to brush my teeth? I can't believe that you tell Dad to brush my teeth so often. I like to have shiny teeth, but the brushing isn't my favorite.

    How is school doing? Are you as good a student as you are a teacher? You need to tell all your friends and teacher about how you help me learn to sit and walk slowly. I know they will be very proud of you. I am!

    I can't wait to see you next week. Where are we going to go on our walk? I heard you guys talking about having a pizza party when you are here. Hopefully I am invited. I love pizza, especially the crust. I promise to behave, but if you drop a few pieces, I will be in heaven!

    Well, I will let you go now. Have a great week at school.

Always remember that like me, you are great girl! You have a friend in me.

From your friend and loyal student,

Magic

Graduation

My Dear Pal:

Congratulations. It's hard to believe that your big day is right around the corner. I am so excited for you. You have worked very hard to get to this point. You need to cherish these moments and celebrate your accomplishments. Over the years I have watched you grow up to become a fine young man. I decided to write this card for the gang of four-leggers because I know I am your favorite. I always enjoy when you come over and I get treated like the Queen, which we know I am! PJ may be the princess but I am the Hartzeneger. I know that I may be buff, but I have the heart of gold.

It seems like yesterday since I graduated as a guide dog puppy in training. I remember having to go off to guide dog school. It was a big step for me. I was scared and lonely, but I promised to do my best. I worked hard but I didn't finish my official dog training because they discovered I had a heart murmur. I was a little disappointed that I couldn't finish off, but honestly I was happy to go home. I missed everyone! I remember how proud everyone was over the accomplishments I had achieved. I guess graduations are big deals for both two- and four-leggers. The real question is, "What have you really graduated from?" Learning is an everyday experience. Although you may have finished high school, you still have a lot more to learn about. Life and growing up will now be your teachers.

I'm writing this letter to you because I've enjoyed watching you grow up to become such a fine young man. You have many talents not only as an athlete but as a kind human being. I sense your kindness because every time I see you, you always make a point to make me feel great. I figured I would use this chance to give you a few of my own "bark insights" on life.

Probably the most important lesson is to always keep your nose on track. You've got to be ready to find unusual

134

scents that may lead you to discover new things. Life isn't about what you know and what you have, but what you can discover and what you can find. Never give up looking for things. Always be inquisitive and try to discover things about yourself and others.

You have had to work hard at your schoolwork, and also to be the best football player you can be. You should never take for granted your God-given talents, because you can lose them in a blink of an eye. Continue to work hard on things that are important to you, but also on things that also may be hard. Life isn't always about winning, but about how hard you work to get to that point. I know that everyone is always excited for those who win, or those who are the best, but I really feel that doing your best is more important. Winners and hard workers, are those people who don't take for granted what they can do, but put forth their best effort. Always remember that you need to do the best you can. It's the man in the glass who you have to look at every day and say "I did what I could and I am proud of it!"

One thing that you know about me is that I like to have a good time. When I get excited you know that I'm happy because my body shakes as I dance the doggy samba. I may look silly, but you've got to celebrate the moments. Seize the day and love it. Life is too short to feel sad. Enjoy the experience! Appreciate what you have while you have it. I know how much you like playing football, and my only suggestion for you is to make sure that while you're playing have lots of fun!

Always try to have a sense of humor. Wagging your tail always lets people know that you're in a good mood. One thing I've learned is you always like to be around people that are happy rather than lumps on a log. I know that you are a fun two-legger. Make sure that others see that fun side in you. They'll want to be around you!

When you leave school behind, I know you won't miss all the homework and things that you're given to do. School has been hard for you and that is OK. There are many things that are hard for me, but I've learned that sometimes digging for bones or working hard at opening a closet will eventually lead me to my rewards(especially when I don't get caught and I get to eat the snack). Sometimes I hear you and Dad (Dr. Fine) *talk about not making excuses about your work. I know it's easy to sometimes put the blame on others (I sometimes try to blame PJ or Magic for the messes that I cause), but eventually I get caught and I pay the price. Learn from your experiences! Take responsibility for your work and actions. No one ever said that life would be totally easy.*

Well, you can see I have a lot to wish for you on your special day. Graduations aren't really endings but new beginnings. I can only wish that on the road to your new beginning that you will celebrate and enjoy all of your life's happenings. I'm so happy for you and I know that even as you become an older two-legger, you'll always have time for me. Congratulations on your big day, Buddy! I am proud of you. Here's a woof for you.

Your pal,

Hart

Death

My dear friend:

I wanted to write you this card to let you know how sorry I was to hear about the death of your father. All of us wanted to tell you that we feel for your loss. I know how important your dad was to you and I know how greatly he will be missed.

I know it may feel weird for you to read a card written by a dog, but I had to do this. I have known you most of my life and you have always been kind to me. You even got me a present on my first birthday. I still have that toy in the house. Your devoted attention and gentle teasing have allowed me to feel loved and wanted by you. You are strict when we walk if I pull you, but I know you just want me to be a more re-laxed walker. Being my friend is what is important. That is a big deal to me; I guess you have been one two-legger that has shown me the true meaning of friendship. Friends are those animals that will stand by you in good times and bad times. Sure, it is fun to hang out with people when things go right, but we need friends when we feel alone and are struggling. This is one of those times where having a friend to talk to or give you a lick is important. I may not talk human, but I am a great listener. Anytime you want to vent out your feelings, call or just come by. We can walk and I will listen, or you can

136

just talk and I will lie by your side. The bottom line is I will be here for you if you want!

You know I haven't ever experienced the loss of a parent, so I don't know exactly how you are feeling. When my brother Shrimp died several months ago, I was very sad. I knew something was different the morning I woke up and he wasn't around. I missed his company. Sometimes my big brother didn't give me the most attention, but knowing he was here was enough. He was my family. There has not been a day that I still don't think about him. Sometimes I even walk by where his food dish used to be, thinking of all the good days we had and how he let me swipe some of his food that he didn't finish. You know me, love those extra treats, but I do need to watch my figure.

Your dad left you with so many great memories. Although his life was taken early, we have to remember all those times and cherish them. Boy, I could hear you now telling me about all the times he took you and the family off roading. They sounded like a lot of fun. Your dad was quite a guy! He loved to spend time with all of you. I know in listening to him talk, that he was very proud of his little boy. He saw your greatness and believed in you. Although he is now not here with you physically, his spirit surrounds you and has become part of your soul. Your dad taught you values and morals, and those beliefs will continue to live on.

Things will be different in your home without your dad. I know it will be hard and all I am going to ask you is to not give up. Be patient and give things time to heal. Things will feel different and all I can tell you is to talk out your feelings rather than hold them in. Holding them in may make things harder for you. It is ok to have those feelings but how you learn to handle them is crucial. Try and take advantage of talking with others. It is like a balloon being filled with air. To avoid having the balloon burst while you are blowing it up, you may need to let some of the air out. So when you are feeling angry, sad or confused, don't be afraid to open up and talk with someone. You can always come over and walk me. I promise I'll listen.

Well that is all I can say now. You are my buddy and I just wanted to let you know that I am here if you need me. My thoughts and the thoughts of the rest of the gang are with you during your loss. Always remember that your dad will be with you in your heart forever.

Your pal,

PJ

Enlisting in the Armed Service

Dear Soldier Boy:

Your dad called the other day and told us that you made it to your base in one piece. We heard that you had a great going away party. Wish we could have been there! We heard there was a lot of food and nice people. You know us, we were most interested in the food, especially things that may have fallen. Bet you there were even cookies! You know we love them! We were happy you liked our card.

Well, you are off! It is hard to realize that you are now all grown up. Where have all the years gone? Over the years, we have all got to know you. I (PJ) heard that you even had a neat relationship with Puppy —that special golden who became your friend. We were just pups when we first met you (except for Shrimp). You were always very nice to us! Holding us when we were younger and always giving us attention every time you came in. We felt important, and I am sure that the attention we gave you showed you the same. In fact, we remember how helpful you were at our birthday party, managing the café, and making sure all our pals got snacks. We really appreciated it when you accidentally (ha ha) dropped a few hot dogs on the ground and we snatched them up, without anyone noticing.

We wanted to send you this special letter to wish you good health and luck as you enter the armed forces. This is a large step in your life, one that you have looked forward to for a long time. Go into it with a positive attitude. Work hard and not only make others proud of you, but most important, be proud of yourself.

Well Hart, Shrimp, and I wanted to share a few words of wisdom with you. Although we may be dogs, we have learned a lot, just by watching people and other animals. Hopefully our little suggestions will be helpful to you.

1. *Kindness cost little but goes a long way. Remember to show your new friends your good side and never be afraid of doing a good deed.*

2. *Be a good person. This is something that everyone has tried to show you.*

3. *Good things are worth working for—we know you know this. Work hard and make things happen!*

4. *People like being around those who have a positive outlook. A positive attitude breeds a healthy lifestyle.*

5. *Success in life is finding out what is important to you. Reach for your stars and grab onto your dreams.*

6. *Appreciate what you have, not what isn't yours. You have so many assets and people who care for you. Cherish and appreciate what you have.*

7. *Be safe. Look after others and hopefully they will look after you.*

Well, that is our 25 cents' worth. We will miss you taking us on walks and teasing us.

Do us and yourself proud. Seize the moments and the day. If you get a chance drop us a note from time to time. If you ever need us, we are only a bark away. Looking forward to seeing you one day soon.

> *Wags, your pals,*
>
> *PJ, Hart, Shrimpy*

On Marriage

Dear friend,

What wonderful news! First finishing school and secondly on getting married! You always made me feel important. I always loved taking our walks. You were always nice to me.

Well, this is your big day! I could say my puppy has grown up, but it is hard to say that, especially because I am still a little girl myself. But while I have been a puppy therapist (mainly working with kids), you are the first to get married on my watch. You now have a new family in the south, and lots of people to look after. I don't have any experience in marriage, but I do have some suggestions on building a family. Family is the most important thing in a dog's life. We live by the rule of the pack, and now you are heading a new one. Remember that a strong pack, or in your case a solid marriage, depends on what you put into it. Make sure you both work hard at it. Don't take it for granted! Let me give you a couple of other bones' worth of insights:

1. *Learn to be a giver, rather than just a taker. It is neat to be needed. I know your wife will look forward to having your loving support.*

2. *Build a life between the two of you. That is what is important. The toys and all the physical things you can buy may be great to have, but having a life built with love and happiness is what you need. Time spent learning to get to know each other and learning to respect each other will make your marriage even stronger.*

3. *Find fun in the relationship. Even in tough times, we need to find that silver lining. Let me tell you one thing. I know what fun is! Work hard but make time to enjoy!*

4. *Keep on the path of your dreams. Doing it with someone you love makes it more rewarding!*

Well, I am going to let you go. I hope you'll have time to drop me and the Doc a note from time to time to let us know how you are doing. We are only a BARK away. It was good to see you again.

Your pal

PJ

Lifting the Spirits of a Friend in Need

This letter was written to a good friend who was going to have surgery. Since we're both dog lovers, it seemed fun and appropriate to have PJ send her best wishes.

Dear Uncle Ron:

I wanted to wish you good luck on Monday. I have my paws crossed that your surgery will go well! I don't actually understand what surgery is, but Dad told me it is a big deal. It is like when I have to go to the veterinarian for some work. Let me tell you, I am a chicken when it comes to going there. Whenever I know that I am going for a visit, it is hard to get me out of the house and even harder to get me out of the car. Last

140

week I wanted to run away from the veterinarian's office when we pulled in. Dad was really smart this time and had my leash right on me. I may be golden, but I am yellow like a chicken. I can't believe that Dad would put me through such torture. He says it isn't for torture at all, but just to help me. I know he would never put me in harm's way, but I need a lot of convincing and reassuring! I think we all do, don't you? He uses a couple of cookies and a quick few pats, to persuade me things will be OK. By the way, what kind of dog biscuits do you like? They sure can make you feel better.

Sometimes not knowing what to expect or being in a new place makes me feel anxious. I may want to run out of the veterinarian's office before he even meets me, but once it is over, I usually walk out with my head held high and my tail wagging. "That wasn't as bad as you thought it would be," I say to myself. I know that is what you will be saying too next week!

Take my advice, uncle, "Be a brave two-legger!" Always remember, "If not now, when? This needs to be done and it will be fine. Things work out for the best. You really need to take care of yourself, so you will be able to get about easier. I promise you when I see you, we can play chase, and I will even let you catch me. When you get home from the hospital you have Loretta and Teddy to take care of you. They won't let you sit still for too long. As for me, I am only a bark away.

I am learning that in life there are things that you have to do that make you feel uncomfortable. You need to have a healthy attitude and think positively. By the time you know it, it will all be over and you'll be home running around. I wish I could tell you this in dog (you would say in person), but we don't speak the same language (although I do write well). However, you have my positive wishes. You are a kind two-legger that cares for all creatures, even cats. I hope your surgery goes well and you feel better real soon. Think positively and work hard to get better. There are many people and other creatures rooting, barking, and even meowing for you.
My thoughts will be with you.

All my best.

Your Pal,

PJ

PS—Hart and Magic are rooting for you too.

141

Ron actually responded a couple days later. This is what he had to say to PJ.

Dear PJ,

You may be yellow but you are also very wise. I will try to make you proud. Give a big kiss to all your special family. I know you got help from Aubrey because he is truly a great writer and special friend to all creatures.

Your friend, Ron

Special Correspondence

Artwork and Drawings

Dear Magic,

I like seeing you when I visit the office. Although I like the other dogs, I like playing with you the most, because you mess around a little more. When that happens, you try and look so innocent when Dr. Fine says, "Let's settle down, Magic."

I remember seeing your puppy picture on the wall. I told Dr. Fine I wanted to draw it, because it looked like something hard to do and I wanted to try it. I hope you like your picture. I worked hard on it.

Well I will go now. I want you to know that you are the first dog I have ever written to. It feels weird, but I am happy that I made the drawing.

Your friend,

Stephen

Dear Stephen:

Wow, I am amazed! I look great! You should see Hart, PJ and Shrimp. They are jealous that you didn't draw a picture of them. I always knew I was the cutest, but I won't tell them that. They may get made at me and hide all my toys. I don't want that to happen.

How long did it take you to finish the drawing? Sometimes things that are hard to do don't come easy. I am proud of you that you took your time and did this for me. If you like I will share one of my chew toys with you when we hang out. Let me tell you, I am not the bestest sharer in the world, but anyone

who takes his time like you did deserves it. Don't ask to play with my favorite ball of socks. I may try to steal it back pretty fast.

Your pal,

Magic

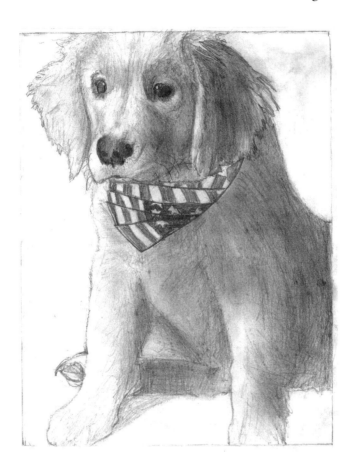

Poems from a Special Friend

Not all correspondence comes in the form of letters. I also receive photos, drawings, and poems. Adrian is a sixth-grade student who has a knack for writing. He has always had a special relationship with all the dogs. In fact, he was the young man who suggested the name Magic for our newest pup. Here are two poems he wrote for Magic and her response to him.

Magic

This new dog Magic
With her soft, gold fur
Can now make a difference
Of the people whose lives are a blur
By taking out the mental fence
And letting them pet her

She got her name a year ago
When me and the Doc were surfin' the net
I gave a few ideas
When we found a name just perfect for his pet
Magic I said
Best name I bet

A year later this cute, furry wonder
Jumps up and down
Play and talk to her
And you'll never frown

We all love dogs
And not one is better than the other
Because they are equal
Like us, one to the other

And not until man loses his friend
Will we understand this miracle
Always till the end
The dog stands near
With a paw to lend
And an understanding ear

The Dog—Our Best Friend

The dog is always near us
He is true and faithful to his master
On the coldest and darkest nights, no fuss
To achieve purpose faster

He guards his master as he sleeps
No one shall pass

144

He licks his master while he weeps
He frolics and plays to make time pass

He never gives up
He's rough and ready
And we look up
To he who is steady

Forever the dog shall remain
To lead or follow
Through joy and pain
Your heart never will be hollow

Dear Adrian:

Wow, you are such a great writer. Thanks for writing both the poems. I really love the one that is named after me. Hopefully when you come by we can go for a good walk. You should show your teacher the poems. I bet she will be as proud of you as I am. Thanks for thinking of me.

Your Pal,

Magic

PJ, Hart, Shrimp, and Magic's Bark Insight

Dear Reader:

We hope you have enjoyed reading some of these notes. Writing has allowed us to let people know that we are thinking of them. It is amazing what this small deed can produce. Receiving letters causes a similar reaction—a smile.

Our suggestion to you is to let people know that they're in your thoughts. Just a simple "Hello, I am thinking about you" may be all that is needed to make friends, family, and co-workers feel better. Writing can also help you express your feelings in a less threatening manner. Perhaps it will be easier for you to write about things, rather than express them in person. Our hope is that you see the value. As it says in the ad, "Reach out and touch someone."

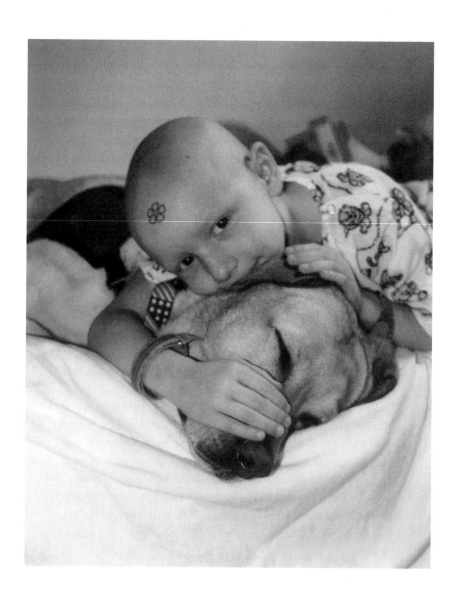

One of Life's Lessons

Carpe Diem

Some may wonder why there is such an intense focus on people and pets in this book. From a purely pragmatic point of view, pets fill a void in most owners' lives. Instead of an empty house, we can come home to a happy dog barking and dancing around for joy that its buddy is home. However, I believe it goes much deeper than that. Many relationships are more than just companionship. Sometimes it is a strong dependency motivated by love. One does not seem to be able to endure without the other, and I hope this book will give more insight into relationships celebrated by poets through the ages.

> *What is love? 'Tis not hereafter*
> *Present mirth hath present laughter,*
> *What's to come is still unsure,*
> *In delaying there lies on plenty*
> *Then come and kiss me sweet and twenty,*
> *Youth's stuff will not endure.*
> (*Twelfth Night* by William Shakespeare)

How can we enjoy the light of day and take from life all that it has to offer if we are alone? There is no joy in loneliness. To live means to love. There are many people who have pets but do not realize the depth of love their pets have for them. Pets have the power to make life worthwhile and utterly memorable. Such is the story of Alexann and Gleason. They symbolize what a powerful effect such devotion can have in someone's life.

This chapter celebrates and remembers those lives. I would like to focus on Alexann's courage and her zest for life in a time that was so hard. We will also focus on a relationship that nurtured her soul and made her last days on this earth more comfortable. Let's meet Alexann and her friend, Gleason.

Lean on Me: I'm Here for You

Framed in the doorway, Alexann lies in the hospital bed hooked up to an IV and the chemotherapy pump. Her six-year-old body looks frail and small among this equipment and bedding; yet she's laughing, cooing and rubbing her bald head in the fur of Gleason, a therapy dog that visits her regularly. Although her condition has weakened, as we look at her there is no doubting or resisting the impish spark in her eyes or that infectious laugh.

This scene reminds us that death is an uncomfortable subject, and as humans we've found any number of ways to justify or rationalize this final step of the life cycle. Case in point, I've just stated one such philosophical view—the pragmatic outlook that all life ends. But there are others, ranging from the cynical—"The only things certain are death and taxes"—to the religious—"She's gone to a better place." With an adult's death, we may find solace in such homilies as "He led a full life" or "At least she died peacefully." But such ideas as these cannot help us with the death of a child. Knowing that those who have left us have not had the chance to experience all that life has to offer often leaves us empty and wondering about the great cosmic plan. Why?

Most often, death leads us to think about what will never be rather than what was accomplished. The death of a child reminds us that there will never be experiences such as a first kiss, learning to drive, or going to college. The other half of this outlook is what the parents and family will never experience—another hug, reading another bedtime story, prom-night photos, or grandchildren.

That we must grieve for our loss is irrefutable. But we can also learn to look at death as not only the closing of a chapter, a loss (a negative), but also as a way to celebrate that life (a positive). Each life, however brief, can teach us about joy if we acknowledge and highlight even the smallest moments.

This brings us back to Alexann, a child who taught those around her that any day can bring a giggle as well as a tear and that both are worth remembering and celebrating. This is a story of determination and a story of friendship. It is a tale of compassion and commitment. The story is of a girl named Alexann and a therapy dog named Gleason, and how Alexann found her greatest happiness in four legs and large, luminous brown eyes.

Sue and her therapy dog, a five-year-old yellow Labrador retriever named Gleason, had been visiting the pediatric ward of a local hospital in Oregon for a year when they first met Alexann in July of 2002. Alexann was six years old, diagnosed with bone cancer, and just beginning chemotherapy when the two met.

When Gleason first walked into her room, Alexann looked over and exclaimed quickly, "Oh! I love dogs. Can he come up on the bed?" Gleason looked to Sue for the okay, and once a blanket was placed on the bed, he hopped up. Alexann gave him a big hug, and a relationship was kindled in that first moment.

Alexann loved animals and had affectionate relationships with her pets, a cat and a dog. She thought of her pets as playmates, and they never resisted, letting her do whatever she wanted, even if the playfulness was silly. Alexann's and her family's lives were turned upside down once she was diagnosed with cancer. In the hospital she had to leave her normal life, which included leaving her beloved pets. Having Gleason around allowed her to find love and security in a difficult and perhaps frightening place. From the moment they met, they were to become soul mates of a sort. Her mom, Wendy, says that when the two met "Something magical took place, and from the first moment there was an immediate connection." Wendy never thought that her daughter couldn't survive, but, as she states, it was as though "Gleason knew what Alexann's destiny was going to be."

From the moment of her birth, Alexann was an exuberant child, always smiling and self-assured. "She should have been a little boy," says Wendy. "Instead of Barbies, she preferred mud and dirt; she liked jeans over dresses."

While she had the strength, Alexann and Gleason would walk the hospital corridors, visiting other children, and Alexann was as playful as ever. One time during a hospital stay, Wendy was preparing Alexann for a shower. "I turned my back for a moment, and she was gone." Then she heard her daughter's laugh and went to the door. Alexann was running stark naked down the hallway, IV pole and all. Even when confined to a wheelchair, Alexann made the most of every minute.

Alexann would often lead Gleason on walks through her hall, visiting the other children in the ward, and the dog would walk slowly and gently with her, looking at her often as if to ask if he were going too fast. She began chemotherapy in June of that year, and Gleason was there almost every day she had a treatment. A month later, Gleason seemed to notice that all of Alexann's hair was gone. To his surprise, he saw in its place a little transfer tattoo adorning the little girl's head. Alexann didn't seem too distraught over the loss of her hair; she loved to rub her bald head on Gleason's soft ears.

Before Thanksgiving, Alexann had to go north to Portland for surgery. According to Sue, Gleason missed her while she was gone, searching for her in the empty hospital room. Alexann returned finally, but her operation had left her with a large cast around her torso that traveled down her legs. At this point, she had to use a wheelchair to move around, but even this did not dampen her spirits. One day, as she navigated the hospital corridors, she came across a young man who was also in a wheelchair. She sang out, "Hey! You want to race?" She had no chance of winning against his electric wheelchair, but that didn't curb her enthusiasm.

Despite the changes, Gleason saw Alexann as the same girl, one with a big smile and even bigger dimples. When she was released from the hospital, Alexann came to visit Sue and Gleason at Sue's home soon after her return from Portland. Once she got there, she horsed around with Sue and her husband, but eventually she gravitated closer to her pal Gleason. She lay down with Gleason on the floor and kissed his ears. He licked her right back. Happy and content with each other, the two fell asleep on the spot.

About a month later, Sue took Alexann and Gleason to a special shop where they could paint pots to give to Alexann's parents as Valentine's Day gifts. On her head, Alexann wore a wig and a hat. She had already mastered the wheelchair, zooming around at top speeds, so this excursion posed no problems. But when the three entered the shop, it was full of kids, all of whom went quiet upon seeing Alexann in her wheelchair. It seemed that they were all a little shocked and curious.

Gleason sat down next to Alexann and, with his presence, became a kind of bridge for the other children to use in approaching her. As children came over to pet Gleason, they struck up a conversation with Alexann. "He is real friendly, you guys, and he loves being around lots of kids. You can pet and hug him. He loves that." As Gleason worked his magic, everyone quickly became comfortable together, seeing Alexann as just another kid (with a very cool dog). As time went on, Alexann even felt secure enough at the pottery store to take off her itchy wig and her hat. With the help of Gleason she felt more at home, and her mom and dad would cherish their Valentine's gifts forever. They would also cherish that day as one where their daughter could be just a kid on the "outside," away from illness and hospital routines and rules.

Even at home, between hospitalizations, Gleason was with her frequently. Alexann and Gleason had formed a special relationship. When at home, Alexann shared photos of him and told "Gleason stories" to her friends and relatives. Wendy remembers, "From the first moment Alexann met Gleason, there was an intimate bond."

Over the next couple of months, things were looking up for Alexann. The medical staff thought her cancer was responding to chemotherapy and all was well. Unfortunately, they were mistaken, and near the end of April Alexann suffered a relapse. She was readmitted to the hospital, and her prognosis worsened. Lying in her hospital bed, she didn't want Gleason to leave for one second. It was as if Gleason was her lifeline, and if she lost him, it would be more than she could endure. Unfortunately, as the disease spread, Alexann had to leave to go to Portland for emergency care. She argued relentlessly to have Gleason join her on her trip, but her arguments were fruitless. This trip she'd be without her dearest companion. Instead, Sue brought Alexann a stuffed yellow Lab so that in some way, Gleason could always be with her.

When Alexann came back from Portland, Sue and Gleason were right there to greet her. Sue states, "I could see in her eyes the pain she was now carrying, but the mere presence of Gleason seemed to lessen it." It was apparent from his slow and gentle movements that he sensed her increasing fragility. A few days later, when he came to visit her, he was afraid of jumping up on her air mattress. He had done this countless times before, but on this day, for the first time, he seemed apprehensive that his big body would hurt the young girl. Sue says, "He looked at me trying to get a better understanding of what he should do next, so I lifted him up onto the bed to be with her. He seemed to know she was dying and wanted to use his warmth and size to keep her comfortable and safe."

After this trip to Portland, Alexann's parents knew in their hearts that they had to tell her she was going to die. Wendy told her that she would be going to heaven, where she would have wings and be free from pain. "If you want to go so bad, why don't you go first? I'm not going anywhere. I am not going to heaven and I'm not going to be an angel," Alexann countered. Whenever someone tried to raise the topic with Alexann, she would ask, "How do you know it's for sure?" This was always followed by, "I don't want to talk about it. We don't have to listen, do we, Gleason?" She refused to give in to the idea of her impending death, regardless of what she was told heaven had to offer.

Then one day, Sue was sitting with Alexann on her hospital bed. The room was filled with balloons and toys from her favorite show, *Sponge Bob Square Pants*. In the room was a big new TV, which Alexann had been given by the Make-A-Wish Foundation when she wished for a "TV bigger than my dad's." Alexann held a blanket adorned with the words "Little Angel," which had become her nickname in the hospital. When Sue and Gleason came to visit that day, Sue decided not to say anything about Alexann's deteriorating health but instead just started to talk to her about her previous dogs. She began to tell Alexann about Big Kahuna and Casey Marie, both of whom had passed on several years before. Sue talked about how she missed her old dogs and how they were in a better place right now. Alexann opened her eyes. She looked at Sue and said, "You never told me that, thanks." After this, she began to accept her death, yet she continued to celebrate every moment of life with smiles and laughter in the company of Gleason.

In the last weeks of her life, Alexann's condition continued to deteriorate. These were hard days for Alexann and her family. For the last six weeks or so, Alexann's parents stayed with her in the hospital day and night, and her sister was there during the last four days.

Aside from her immediate family, Sue and Gleason saw Alexann more than anyone else. In the two weeks before she died, she lost feeling from her waist down and was in a light coma. But when Gleason hopped onto her bed, and her hand was placed on him, she would pet him and even give him a small smile. Sometimes Alexann's fingers would cover his nostrils, but he didn't budge except to open his mouth to breathe. Sue says, "He loved that girl, and she loved him." When Sue told Gleason it was time to go, he refused to leave Alexann's side. He scooted closer to her and licked her face. Sue had to physically pull him off the bed. Before he was finally removed from the bed, Gleason licked her hand for the final time.

Later that evening, Alexann died. It was Wednesday, May 28, three days before her seventh birthday. When Wendy called Sue to let her know that she had died, Gleason began to howl, even before she went over to him. Sue remembers, "He was inconsolable that evening and howled for two hours."

A memorial service was held one week after Alexann's death. Sue and Gleason attended, along with many of the pediatric nurses from the hospital. Projected on an 8 × 10-foot screen was a picture of Alexann and Gleason. There was even a pew reserved for them. The sign read: "For Gleason, the Wonderful Therapy Dog." Gleason's presence at the service was soothing to many. Even Alexann's little sister wanted Gleason around her all the time and took him for a walk around the church. Like all who attended that day, Gleason was there to commemorate the life of his friend—a friend he stood with until the day she left.

During the service, many people shared how Alexann had touched their lives. One of her doctors spoke of her effect on the whole hospital ward, and Alexann's mother read a letter she'd written to her daughter. Remarkably, a woman who barely knew Alexann told how the young girl had saved her life. During their return trip from Portland, she and her parents stopped at a restroom. In the bathroom, Alexann met a woman who, unknown to Alexann, had just been diagnosed with cancer. She was inspired by this small girl's bravery and spirit. She then revealed that she had been planning to commit suicide. If not for this brief encounter with Alexann, she would have shot herself that very day.

Following the service, one hundred red (Alexann's favorite color) balloons were released to symbolize her free spirit and celebrate the mark she left on those who had known her. Everyone who met Alexann had been touched by her exuberance and zest for life. As Sue states, "There was some kind of light that exuded from her . . . she changed my whole life."

Sue says that Gleason knows Alexann is in a better place. He can now pass by her hospital room without looking for her but says that the "little angel" lives on in the heart of Gleason and the many others who loved her.

Wendy says she cannot put into exact words Alexann's relationship with Gleason. "He was the only sunshine that lifted her spirits whenever she was in the hospital." Gleason was not only a comfort to her daughter but also to Wendy. She knew that if she couldn't be there, Gleason would be. "Alexann was in good 'paws' with Gleason by her side. I know she is in heaven waiting for her friend and companion."

Wendy remembers the day of the memorial service as a typical Oregon gray one. But what she remembers best is a brief moment when the clouds parted and a shaft of sunlight shone down. "This is how I'll remember her—a memorable moment in my life. She brought us joy."

Although Alexann's life was short, she blessed all those around her. Life's blessings are more than daily prayers and rituals. Blessings are events that make a difference in our lives. Alexann's life was a blessing to her family and to those she touched. Death brings a feeling of loss, but we can work through these feelings if we celebrate the life lived—if we seize every moment as precious. Bryan Mellonie wrote a very touching children's book called *Lifetimes,* where he explains death. Every life has a noticeable beginning and ending. Some lives are longer, and some are shorter. But between these two points are moments of joy and sadness, and each one is valuable. Mellonie emphasizes that this is our "lifetime." No matter the length of time we stay, it is the remembering and celebrating of the "middle" that we should emphasize. What we need to hold on to are the memories that enrich our souls. We should preserve these memories as everlasting tributes to those who die. As we share these "middle" events, the life that has ended can continue to live in giving of itself to others.

Hart's Bark Insight

Life is all around us. All we have to do is recognize that it is. I love cool mornings with heavy dew on the grass. I love to tug on Aubrey's pant leg as he drinks coffee and gazes out the window. I like to remind him that the world awaits just outside the door. I like to think that the other animals and I help him remember to celebrate each day as a new beginning, to smell the life all around him. Although I mark the same bushes and trees as the night before, I never tire of putting my nose to the test over and over, for each time brings something new. For me, each day is treated as a new challenge. I especially like the sheer joy of being alive and on the move—smelling, running, playing and barking. It is the present that counts, and if I find a surprise along the way, the day is all the more exciting. So pick the grape and drink the wine. Live today as if tomorrow will never come. This is the lesson Alexann teaches us—grab life moment by moment, embrace both the tears and the giggles.

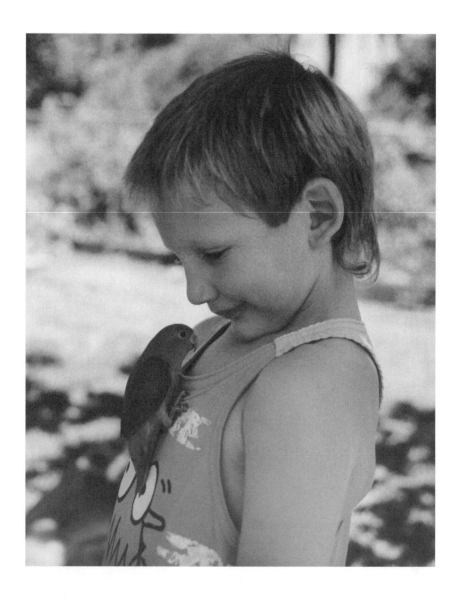

Remembering Lifetimes

> *Grieve not, nor speak of me with tears, but laugh and talk of me as if I were beside you. . . I loved you so— 'Twas heaven here with you.*
>
> —Isla Paschal Richardson

When Corey graduated from elementary school, his teacher asked all the students to write a thank-you letter to their parents.

> *Dad: No matter what happened and what my problem was, you were there for me! Remember when Coshi died and you were supposed to give a speech but you stayed home and comforted me? We read a story, drew a picture and buried my good pal. Dad, you cried with me, laughed with me and cared for me. Thank you Dad — I love you. Corey*

The death of Coshi impacted all of us. Sixteen years have gone by and we still talk about this beloved pet. I smile every time I hear Corey reflect on his relation with Coshi. We still have a picture in the living room of the two of them. We cannot alter the course of events, but we can always cherish what we had. That is what this chapter does; it celebrates, cherishes what we have had. Most importantly, it shows us how to embrace and give meaning to these lives so that our own are enhanced.

Although my first personal experience with the loss of an animal stems back to Sasha's death, it is the vivid memory of my son's pet bird that has helped me realize the importance and value of celebrating life.

In 1989 Corey adopted a beautiful peach face love bird that we named Coshi. The bond between the two of them was remarkable. Corey was only in preschool at the time, and over a few short few months, they formed a solid bond.

Wherever Corey went, the bird tagged along, hanging onto his shirt. I used to get a kick out of watching Corey come to the kitchen in the morning with Coshi dangling from his pajama top. It was a sight to see. We even called some of his shirts "Coshi's shirts" because they were slightly chewed around the neck. Yet my rambunctious young pre-schooler was always gentle with the tiny bird. They were great playmates, something we don't associate with a boy and a bird.

One of my favorite memories is how he would drive her around in his small Batmobile car. They were a real pair. Imagine watching Corey push this tiny bird in a toy car. He always placed her on the seat of the vehicle and slowly pushed her around the floor. "Varoom! Varoom! Here we go, Coshi." She would gaze out the window as the Batmobile rolled throughout the house. Even though Corey sometimes pushed the car out to the driveway, Coshi stayed put. Interestingly, Coshi took the role of the Caped Crusader, and Corey was Robin. What a very different Dynamic Duo, but one that worked well.

During an early afternoon in October of 1991, a tragic event occurred. Corey was playing with Coshi outside in the backyard. As he did on numerous occasions, he sat on the grass while he gently tossed her in the air. Coshi loved fluttering back down into his lap. Unfortunately, the unexpected happened. Out of nowhere an eager cat pounced, and in a moment, Corey's friend was in his grasp. All Nya could hear from the backyard was Corey shouting for help. He was hysterical and in tears, and by the time Nya rescued Coshi, it was too late. What an awful sight for Corey to witness! He had seen his good friend die and had been unable to rescue her.

Nya called me immediately, and as I rushed home, all I could think of was what tremendous pain Corey must be going through. Not only was he mourning the loss of Coshi but also dealing with the guilt that he had, perhaps, caused her premature death. Once I arrived, we sat in silence for a while, and then suddenly we were both in tears. I knew it was going to be hard to explain to a young child what had happened to Coshi, but I also knew we needed to talk about it. Corey had never experienced death, but today he had been forced to see a more brutal side of life. I decided that taking a drive would be a good idea. We drove to the nearby park and continued to talk. "Why, Dad, why did this have to happen?"

he asked with a shaky voice. "I hate that cat; he should have never done that to her." Corey needed to get these feelings out, so I just sat and listened because any comment I made wouldn't erase what had happened. I listened for the next twenty minutes as he told and retold the story. He looked so lost and mournful that I thought my own heart would break.

I suggested to Corey that we go to the park, away from the house, which, in Corey's young mind, was the "scene of the crime." Before I'd left my office, I had gathered a couple of children's books about the loss of a pet. I thought they might be helpful in getting Corey to open up. After the worst of the crying was over, he sat quietly as I read the first story. Although he was still crying softly, he concentrated on listening to it. After reading the story, we talked a bit more, and then I suggested Corey draw a picture of Coshi and himself as Batman and Robin. Coshi never looked better as Batman. The exercise of drawing temporarily distracted Corey from his misery so that we could talk about the practical side, where we could bury his bird. Corey suggested a shaded place in our backyard. He also wanted a monument to mark the spot, so before we drove home, we stopped at a local masonry shop and purchased a small bird bath.

We wrapped Coshi in a yellow cloth and placed her in a small box. The next day we buried her. Corey helped dig the grave, and we had a short ceremony as the whole family stood around the plot. Corey was the last to bid farewell, and he said a special prayer for her. Then Corey gently placed the box into the ground as tears flowed from his eyes. He began to shovel dirt into the tiny hole, determined to complete this task without our help. On that day in October, my little boy grew up a little bit more. For the first time in his life, he experienced loss. It was hard for him to accept, but what kept him going were all the wonderful memories he had. Over the weeks that passed, Corey and I spent a great deal of time talking about Coshi's lifetime and all the joy they had brought each other. Memories would never bring back her life, but celebrating the love made it easier for him to cope.

The sad part about any life is that for many, it ends too soon. What we hold on to are the memories that enrich us. We preserve these memories as everlasting tributes. We remember and celebrate the moments we once had together. Carl Sandburg offered this thought: "Life is like an onion. You peel it off one layer at a time, and sometimes you weep." We weep for our loss and a life that no longer exists. On the other side, we also can rejoice in a life lived. This chapter discusses these aspects of death—weeping, rejoicing, celebrating and remembering.

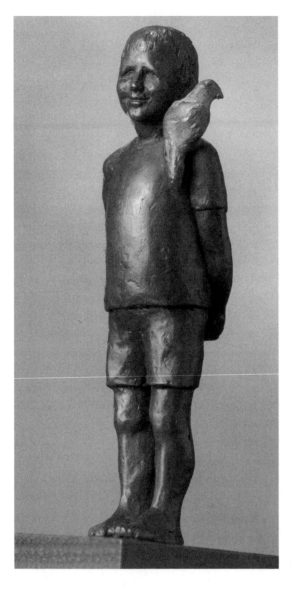

Corey and Coshi

I can only imagine the pain Alexann's parents have endured since the death of their daughter. However, I have witnessed the effects of a child's death. In 1982, a few months after the birth of my first son, Sean, I received a phone call from my mother-in-law, letting me know that my sixteen-year-old sister-in-law, who suffered from a severe developmental disability, had died. I dreaded going home to tell Nya about her sister. I can still visualize the moment. There she sat with Sean in her arms, calling out, "Look who's here! Daddy is home to play with you." Only a few moments later, her extreme joy turned into overwhelming sorrow. This death was hard on the entire family, but especially on Nya's parents. For them, Lisa's death was devastating. Lisa's care had filled their hours from morning 'til night. With her death, the parents were left with not only the loss but also a great void. What would they do? How would they pass these empty hours? These questions, along with others, had to be answered during the healing process.

Growing up a member of a traditional Jewish family in Montreal, the celebration of the High Holy Days was always a big deal. My mother and grandparents would prepare for weeks to usher in the Jewish New Year, the first of the holidays. Special foods were bought in and the dining room table was all dressed up with fine china and flowers. According to my grandparents, the New Year, Rosh Hashanah, required preparation. It symbolized a fresh start, and so the holy day is ushered in like royalty. Yom Kippur, the Day of Atonement, follows ten days later. Yom Kippur means "Day of Atonement" and it is on this day that we repent for the sins of the past year. Theologians tell us that it is on Yom Kippur that God inscribes all of our names in the book of life and the judgments entered in these books each year are sealed, never to be changed.

The Jews of Montreal form a unique community that has a strong cultural life. Unlike many other large Jewish cities, Montreal's ties have preserved its European heritage, and the practices today are a direct reflection of tradition. Jewish community life in that city hasn't changed in decades. My childhood experiences were similar to thousands of Jewish children who lived in "shtetils" of the old country. Although the way of life has changed, the community itself is still well-insulated. What can I tell you? The High Holy Days were a big deal, much different from my life today as an assimilated Jew residing in Los Angeles.

My first experience with the death of an immediate family member was my grandfather, who died only a few days before Yom Kippur, the Jewish Day of Atonement. Therefore, my feelings for this solemn holiday were transformed some decades ago. Tradition requires a Jew be buried very quickly after his or her death. Knowing my grandfather would have wanted me at his service, the family agreed to hold the funeral until the day after Yom Kippur. I remember flying home the eve of the Holy Day with tears in my eyes. I sat on the plane writing a eulogy about my grandfather. My "Zayda," as I called him, was my surrogate father. My mom and dad separated when I was quite young, and my grandparents took on great responsibilities in my upbringing. I believe that because my grandfather was blind we became even closer. He depended on me to help him out, and these needs made our relationship stronger.

The next morning I went to the synagogue for the Holy Day service, but I couldn't concentrate on the prayers of repentance. My mind kept wandering to my grandfather. When I was a boy, I always accompanied him to the synagogue. I would help him find his seat, and when the service finished, I would walk him back home. As I stood in the synagogue on that day, all I wanted was to be that boy again. Instead of hearing the prayers, I heard his voice.

During the Yom Kippur service a time is designated to honor the souls of the departed. The memorial service is known as Yizkor, which means "remembrance." The Yizkor service is celebrated four times a year. On Yom Kippur it is couched between the morning and afternoon services. Tradition excuses congregants from the service if they don't have any departed loved ones. When I was a child, the Yizkor service was like an intermission, or the seventh-inning stretch. It was an excuse to go out and mingle. Often I would skip out with my buddies, sometimes not returning to the synagogue for a couple of hours. The Yom Kippur of 1983 would be different. I stayed for the Yizkor service. For the first time, I recited the mourner's Kaddish, a memorial prayer in memory of those of who have died. I looked around the synagogue that morning and saw many people with tears in their eyes. Now I was joining them. In the space of thirty-six hours, I had grown up and faced a new adversary: death.

The Holy Day of Yom Kippur has not been the same since my grandfather's death in the fall of 1983, and his passing so close to the holy day has changed my view of it. This holy period is no longer associated with ushering in the New Year and making a fresh start in repenting slights and sins; instead, I remember my loss. I don't think this is necessarily unhealthy, but it is vastly different from my joyous childhood experiences. Back then, I could have never fathomed that my feelings of loss would be repeated under similar circumstances in the future.

Yizkor: Remembering Puppy

I use the story of my grandfather's death to segue into discussing the demise of Puppy. Puppy started to show significant signs of aging by the end of 1999. She tired more easily and was often found napping in my office. She had aged gracefully, and my "girlfriend" was now a beautiful "grand dame."

Although Puppy had never seemed threatened by the younger Hart's involvement in my practice, she would upstage Hart. Hart would enthusiastically greet the patients at the front door. When things had quieted down, Puppy would make her entrance to let Hart know she was still in command. It was fun to watch, but I could tell that Puppy was having a hard time letting go of her primary role as a therapy dog. I thought of retiring her a few times, but the sight of her standing at the door waiting to leave for the office was too hard to ignore.

Thursday, October 5 was a tough day. When we arrived home from the office she vomited. I sat with her the whole evening trying to get her to drink a little. By the morning, she looked a little perkier but definitely not herself. It turned out that Thursday was her last afternoon at the office. Although she didn't move around too much, her appetite was good for the next couple of days. My hopes for Puppy's recovery were now more real; I knew these were her final days, and I just wanted to hold on, to cheat death.

On the eve of Yom Kippur, Puppy had a rough night and couldn't keep much food or water down, but in the morning she roused herself and went outside. A short while later Nya became concerned and went to check on her. Like many ill animals, Puppy had removed herself from the pack to find a pleasant spot in the yard where she could be alone. When I went over to her, I could see her discomfort. She reeked from the smell of new vomit that covered her fur. She looked pitiful. She had lost her glow and in many ways, her spark of life. When I saw her, I lay next to her for a few moments, gently stroking her head and trying to say a few kind words but it was too much for me. I began to weep.

I decided to carry her back into the house and gently placed her on the floor. Nya came over and we started to give her a warm sponge bath. She looked hopeless but seemed to appreciate our efforts. She also seemed to feel better now that the stench was removed from her fur (or at least we did). Nya placed a phone call to the veterinarian. I stroked Puppy's head for a while as I began to dry her fur. Nya came back and took over for a few moments while I went to the refrigerator to get Puppy a few ice chips. I had just left the room when Nya called, "We're losing her." I ran back and placed Puppy's head in my lap, and in just a few moments, she was gone. I cried like a baby.

It was Yom Kippur, another Day of Atonement—another year when death paid a visit, as it had seventeen years before to my grandfather, and as I did so many years earlier, I went to the synagogue that morning with a feeling of emptiness and a bruised heart.

Years after Puppy's death, while I have healed, her legacy still shines in my heart as well as in the "souls" of my other therapy dogs. Puppy was my first real animal co-therapist, and I credit her with invoking my passion with animal-assisted interventions. My life has been turned around because of our relationship. Puppy brought out a gentle side in me. She brought more laughter and kindness into the workplace.

Puppy's departure was unlike any other death I have experienced. I couldn't mourn in private and I had to tell others of and relive Puppy's death. Every time a client came in, her or his first comment would always be, "Where's Puppy?" Once they were told of her death, I would then have to acknowledge their feelings of loss. Over the course of the month, I received many cards of condolences, from past and present clients. Some children drew pictures of their beloved Puppy while others wrote poems. Here are a few of my favorites.

One eleven-year-old boy spent a weekend writing this poem, which also incorporated a picture he drew of Puppy.

Puppy

Puppy was a gentle dog.
She made me feel relaxed.
She always was insistent.
When it came to petting her.

Puppy was a famous dog.
She made a cool discovery.
That dogs calm down patients.
And make them feel at home.

Puppy is in heaven now.
But had a good life here.
Because Dr. Fine took care of her.
And took her from the streets.

Puppy we will miss you lots.
And so will Shrimp and Hart.
But with happy thoughts we think of you.
We'll remember you a lot.

A nine-year-old girl prepared this poem as her letter of remembrance. It was surrounded by a warm-hearted illustration of Puppy. She writes:

PUPPY

Cute
Friendly
Happy
Gentle
PUPPY

Sweet
Lovable
Soft
Fun
PUPPY

Loves to walk
Excited
Curious
Helpful
PUPPY

We love you, Puppy, we'll miss you!

Finally, this is one of the many notes that I received on her behalf. This was written by an eleven-year-old boy who had known Puppy for several years. He was a quiet and sensitive young boy who enjoyed her company as we sat and talked on numerous afternoons. He shares:

Doctor Fine

I was very sorry that Puppy died. She was a great dog. And my favorite. I used to laugh when you told me funny stories about Puppy. When I found out she died from my sister, I just started to cry. I am very sorry about it, but remember, all dogs go to heaven!

Receiving notes like these helped me, and I felt that I was dealing well with Puppy's death. A few months prior to Puppy's passing, I had agreed to present a lecture at the National Conference in San Francisco on Pets Are Wonderful Support. I had almost finished the entire Power-Point presentation prior to Puppy's death, and many of the slides had pictures of her. I almost cancelled speaking at the conference because I thought it was too soon to share my personal impressions of the value of animal-assisted interventions. However, I decided that if I kept the talk more informational, I could avoid becoming emotional. As I stood before the audience, I was surprised that I didn't feel any emotion when discussing Puppy's contribution to my therapy work. As the lecture progressed, I became more confident that I could share more intimate details. I couldn't have been more wrong.

At the end of the lecture, I decided to tell a story about one young boy named Alex who had been very moved by Puppy's death. I told the audience how I could still see him looking at me and innocently asking, "Will I ever see her again? Is she in heaven, Dr. Fine?" And then he said, "I really hope she is okay. I miss her." I told the audience that at first I was speechless. How to respond? Somehow I managed to pull it together and have a good discussion on death and loss. Alex told me, "She made me feel at home, Dr. Fine, and that is what I will miss the most." I went on and explained to the crowd, as I had to Alex, that Puppy was a blessing. Although he and I would never see her again physically, she would be within our hearts forever. As his eyes filled with tears that afternoon he looked at me and said, "I am happy that I met her. I will miss her a lot. Things will be different around here without her. I will say a prayer for her tonight. I know she is making a new home in heaven." I spoke to my audience of how I knew Puppy's influence on Alex would continue to bless him forever.

It was the word "forever" that did it. For the first time in my professional life, I began to weep in front of my audience. I was so embarrassed about becoming emotional, especially in front of such a large audience, that I looked down at the floor. I had thought I could avoid those emotions. I was hesitant to look back up. What would I see—laughter, pity, and people flying up the aisles in a hasty retreat? But I had to finish; I had to make an exit. I took a deep breath and looked up. No one had left. All of them were sitting quietly, and many were crying right along with me. Death has the power to bond us all together.

On October 19, 2000, I went to San Francisco to give a lecture and was joined by my peers, by other professionals, in holding a memorial service for Puppy. I realize now that I had never truly grieved, that I had put it off in telling only of her death and my effort to comfort my patients during their loss.

I received a great deal of positive feedback from many who attended the workshop. It wasn't until five years later, however, that I realized how much I had touched the audience. While attending another conference in Glasgow, Scotland, I went for a walk. Then I heard my name called. I knew few people in Glasgow, and those I did were still at the conference. When I turned around there was an unfamiliar gentleman standing before me. He introduced himself as a veterinarian who had attended that session many years ago in San Francisco.

After we exchanged pleasantries for a while, he told me, "Your lecture made a real impact on me. As a veterinarian, I have experienced the death of many of my clients, but on that afternoon you put a face and a story behind those animals and what they have done for so many." He then went on to tell me how much he appreciated those words and the emotions that were released in the room. He made it clear that Puppy's life story had also inspired him professionally. I left our brief meeting renewed. Puppy was still an inspiration; her life had meant something. Life has a beginning and an end, but it is the between times, the lifetime, that we should remember. The moments and events between birth and death are what enliven our hearts and souls.

Shrimp: The Legacy Lives On as We Celebrate Life

I have a golfing buddy, Rudi, who loves dogs. Much of our time on the golf course we spend telling dog stories. It was early on Sunday, June 25, and Rudi was telling a "Daisy Story." Daisy, a young beagle, was his mother's dog. Before his mother died, Rudi promised her that he would take Daisy. Over the past months they have bonded. He admitted that their special relationship seemed related to their joint history, his mother.

Like most mornings, we alluded to the antics of our dogs. Rudi had shared briefly that Daisy continued to have traits of Houdini, and loved the challenge of escaping. Just that morning, Rudi had to follow her down the street and give her a "talking to." Rudi is fond of saying that Daisy is the perfect irony for his youthful indiscretions and the pain he caused his mother. But she is a sweet, loving dog who cares for people.

On this morning, we also talked about Shrimp and his continued discomforts in mobility. The past several months had been harder for him to get up on his own. I could almost feel his pain as I watched him. Once on his feet, however, he hobbled around quite well. I had started taking Shrimp on solo walks, since he didn't have the stamina to keep up with the other dogs, and frankly, I enjoyed the slower pace. I told Rudi that I had to chuckle to myself as we took our walk. We looked like two old men by the time we reached home, shuffling at a snail's pace. It didn't seem to bother Shrimp and at the end of our pleasant journey, he seemed content that he had completed the walk as he returned to the office and slowly lowered his body down to the floor.

As Shrimp got older, life's simple pleasures were harder for him to attain. In fact, I have been preparing myself for his eventual passing. This has been going on for months. Only about four months ago, he appeared to be struggling to get to sleep. His breathing was hard, and he seemed uncomfortable lying down. I really thought he was going to die that night. Like a little boy, I quietly crawled out of bed and snuggled next to my buddy. There I was, bundled with my blanket, on the floor comforting Shrimp. My presence seemed to ease his pain, and with gentle strokes on his forehead, he eventually fell asleep. His breathing even became more relaxed.

I told Rudi about one of the first nights that I slept on the floor. Initially, I was not noticed by the rest of the dogs, who were deep in sleep. However, as time passed, PJ noticed where I was and wandered over to lie next to me. In a short while, I was surrounded by my entire group. Even little Magic seemed to understand that calm was needed. At first she was ready to start playing, straddling over me as if I were a huge log. But she sensed quickly that her timing was off, that I was there to make Shrimp more comfortable. We all seemed to be standing guard, a vigil providing Shrimp with the emotional support that we hoped would make him feel better.

While Rudi and I talked about him, I remembered that Shrimp was about to turn fifteen the next day (June 26). All of our younger dogs had a birthday cake given to them on at least one of their birthdays. That had not been the case for Shrimp. I am not quite sure why this happened, but we didn't seem to be that adventurous while celebrating his milestones. Well, I decided, that needed to change.

Rudi lives in Pasadena, quite close to one of the dogs' favorite establishments, the Three-Dog Bakery. Over the years we have ordered numerous cakes and cookies, and I asked Rudi if he would pick up a cake for Shrimp so we could all celebrate his big day in style. Rudi agreed that would be a good thing to do, and he said he would bring it by the next afternoon.

Shrimp accompanied me to work as usual. I was quite excited to get home to mark the special occasion. After dinner, I made a point to take the cake out of the box to photograph it. Once that was done, I left it on the counter and went over to take a few shots of Shrimp, who was lounging in the family room. He has never been a fan of photographs, but he indulged me in posing for a few. I was about to cordon off the kitchen for the celebration, when I looked over my shoulder and saw PJ on her hind legs, hovering over the cake. Discovered by both Nya and

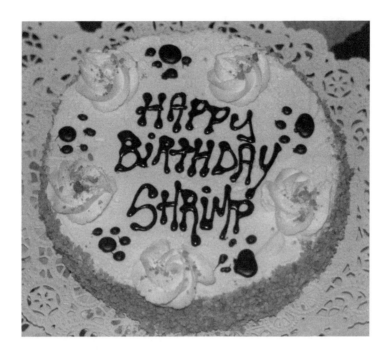

me, she was quickly reprimanded and sent to her room for a time-out. She looked so helpless and innocent as she was escorted to the room by Warden Nya. I am certain PJ wasn't worried that she would miss Shrimp's party but rather of not getting her portion of the cake.

Once we had dealt with the PJ misadventure, I turned my attention back to Shrimp. I helped him get back up and directed him to the kitchen, where I had placed the semi-frosted cake on the floor. When he got closer to the cake, he seemed to ignore its presence, even after my urging. To help him take notice of his new treasure, I scooped some of the frosting onto my finger and let Shrimp lick it off. He eagerly took it all off my finger and patiently waited for round two. We went through this a few more times, before he eventually realized that the cake was there for his devouring. He was ready to dive right in, and what a beautiful sight it was. It took fifteen years for Shrimp to have his first cake, and I wasn't about to deprive him of this moment. He was joined by Hart and Magic, who were eager to get their fair share. There would even be enough leftovers for all of them (including PJ) the next day, but for the moment, it was Shrimp's turn to bask in the limelight. We were there to celebrate his life, not mourn his impending departure. It was a "dog celebration" I would cherish forever. Life is not all suffering and pain. Sometimes the sun breaks through and brings hope and happiness.

The Circle of Life: The End of a Legacy

For the past several months, as I mentioned to Rudi, I had tried to avoid Shrimp's inevitable passing. Shrimp had started life the hard way and was fighting just as hard at the end. As days progressed, it was more and more difficult for him to sleep in comfort. Nya and I took turns spending part of a night lying close to our friend. On Thursday, July 6, Shrimp had had the toughest night ever. He cried in his sleep, letting us know he was in pain. We knew then that would be his last night in our home.

It is amazing how some beings, no matter what their own circumstances, always protect and shield those around them from the harsher realities. This was our Shrimp. When we rested next to him, he seemed to be the comforter, trying to hide his pain for our benefit. We had called the veterinarian and explained our dilemma and set an appointment for that evening. With some help, Shrimp got up a couple of times to go to the bathroom, but by mid-afternoon, he lay on the floor with little movement. It would soon be time for our appointment, but Nya and I decided to leave early.

He hadn't eaten all day, but I thought Shrimp deserved his favorite treat of french fries, even if he could only enjoy the smell. Next we decided to go to my office, Shrimp's home away from home, for one last visit. He looked very helpless as he reclined in the back seat, holding onto his last drop of life. Once at the office, I decided it wasn't fair to him to carry him into the office he loved so much. Nya and I stood in the parking lot commiserating with each other. She had been with Shrimp most of the day and her eyes were as red as a Macintosh apple. Nya has never been afraid of shedding tears, and today was no different. We hugged for a while, and I gave her some time alone with Shrimp, but she knew I had to take Shrimp to the veterinarian by myself.

Once on the road, I talked to Shrimp. I wanted to reminisce with him for the last time. Ironically, just being around him was all I could think about, and this would be what I missed the most, turning around and seeing him in my back seat or looking at him through my rearview mirror, gazing into his beautiful dark eyes. I let him know he was "my best big boy," but I really wanted him to reassure me that I was about to do the right thing. Ending a life, even when we know it will end all the pain, is still hard to do.

We got to the clinic around 7:15 p.m. Once we checked in, we were escorted to Room One. I placed a blanket from home on the floor and gently lowered Shrimp. After about fifteen minutes, I was told there was an emergency and it would be a while until we would be seen. Perhaps on a different occasion, I would have been impatient, but tonight I was in no rush, and the extra time was a blessing.

Twelve years ago, just before his life ended, I read Goldie, my first dog, a book called *I Always Love You* by Hans Wilhelm. The story is beautiful, for it shares the relationship that a boy has with his beloved dog. They had grown up with each other, and when the dog doesn't arise in the morning, the boy finds solace in the fact that he always told his beloved dog that he loved her. As I snuggled next to Shrimp, just like a little boy, I began to read the story to him, putting his name into appropriate places and elaborating about him wherever possible. For example: "Sometimes Nya would get angry with Shrimp when he would dig up a storm, but she loved him, even when he got scolded. We would both tell our little boy, 'We'll always love you.' We knew deep down inside he understood."

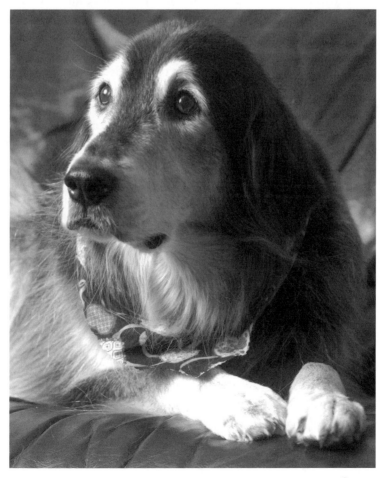

Tears were flowing easily while I read the story. Although I tell all my pets that I love them, I knew this would be the last time I could tell Shrimp in person, and I couldn't say it enough. We cuddled for the next forty-five minutes as I gently stroked his head and back. He didn't want to drink anything, but, while fumbling in my pockets, I realized that I had a few pieces of venison jerky. To my surprise, when I presented it to him, he took it and munched on it. It made me feel more at ease.

The veterinarian finally came in and examined Shrimp. She concurred with Nya and me. There was nothing else we could do. Having the opportunity to be with Shrimp for over an hour, I told her that I would need just a few more minutes. I looked at Shrimp for reassurance and hugged him hard. The veterinarian returned and then explained what she was going to do. I sat next to Shrimp and gently placed his head on my lap. I looked hard in his eyes and for the last time I whispered gently, "I'll always love you." It only took about eight seconds for his heart to stop. I hugged his soft body and cried one more time before leaving. That night I left only with his collar, name tag, and a heart full of wonderful and breathtaking memories. My Shrimp was gone.

As I write this, it has been a couple of months since Shrimp passed away. Not many days go by that I don't think about him. In fact, what I miss the most are some of the little things, like how his claws had a specific rhythm all their own on the hardwood floors. Just as with his mother, Puppy, over the course of about a month I received many letters of condolence from members of Shrimp's fan club. Until then, I never realized how much of an impact he had had on so many people. I knew that he was popular with the older children, but I really didn't recognize just how popular he had become. Here are just a few the notes that I received:

Shrimpy
You'll be so missed! Your quiet strength and sweet temperament were always so welcoming. You always brought a smile to my daughter's heart. She and I will miss you so much. You are the quiet rock of the group.

Shrimp
It only seems to be a disaster when we think you're not here anymore. You were always my favorite because of how relaxed and obedient you were. I know you're still here in our hearts and the dogs' hearts. We will hear your barks in our dreams.
Sincerely,
your friend

Hey Shrimpy:

Gosh, I can't believe you're gone. I've known you since I was a little girl. I bet now you're in dog heaven, Puppy is grooming you like you were little again. Make sure you give Puppy a bark and a tail wag for me, okay? I love you and miss you all.
Always yours,
 your friend.

Shrimps

These days have been good for you. You'll be remembered in all our hearts. Thank you for the calm you brought in these visits. You made it easier for me to open up and talk.
Thanks in love, your friend

Shrimp

You are an amazing dog and a friend to have. You would always make me smile even when I was sad. Coming to the office I would always look forward to see you and hear all the stories about you from Dr. Fine. You are in a much happier place now and definitely will never be forgotten! We never got to go to the prom or homecoming together (as I would tease Dr. Fine, when I initially didn't have a date, and said you were loyal and would be a good choice), but you would have made the other girls jealous. We miss you here with us. We will never forget you, Shrimpy.
Love,

The messages don't make the loss easier to accept, but they do help me realize the importance of Shrimp's lifetime. The lifetime is what we need to hold on to so that the legacy can be preserved. It's only when those memories are forgotten that the soul may be lost.

Here's what I imagine Shrimp would say if he could talk:

Shalom, mien Mentsh,

You didn't know I spoke Yiddish, did you? But after all those years with you and the holy days we spent together, I should have learned something. Those were special years for me. Your touch and your smell will be with me forever. We shared a lot of secret moments, such as our short walks from the office to McDonald's to get some "exercise" and a few french fries. However, I never had to brush my teeth when I got home; I just dug a hole and stuck my muzzle in it. A little dirt goes a long way to cover a lot of sins.

But actually, mien Mentsh, ours was a good life. We shared everything—walks, talks, and baths. Whatever I did, you always encouraged me, guided me and allowed me to help you and those who came to you for help. I was overjoyed, licking and smelling all those wonderful kids. Those were the best days of my life. I loved licking those fresh young faces and listening to them giggle and then hug me. My ears never went without a good scratching every day. Real happiness is being scratched and receiving a secret treat for responding. When the day ended, we headed home, where the rest of the family waited. I loved you all. You all made my life better than a bone fresh from the butcher's. Thanks for the birthday cake, even though it took you fifteen years to remember. I should have peed in your shoe years ago, but the fries kept me in line. I hope you remember Nya's birthday. I won't be there to remind you, so you'd better write it on your paw.

I hate to say goodbye, but when the time comes for you, Puppy and I will be waiting, so we can all run and play in celestial parks just like we used to do. Remember to keep candy for the kids and dog treats for the gang at home.

Ich liebe dich.

Shrimp

The souls of Coshi, Shrimp, and Puppy will never be forgotten. They have become the fabric of the lives they touched. I miss both Puppy and Shrimp, but all I have to do is close my eyes for a moment and see them both next to me. Sure, I am not able to touch them, and I miss holding them. But there is a part of me that knows that their souls are still alive within my heart. I can only be grateful for the time that I had. Thanks for the afternoons!

Hart's Bark Insight

Corey is home for a couple of weeks before he returns to school in the fall. In May of this year he experienced the death of his good friend Ben, who died in an automobile accident. The loss of Ben has devastated Corey, par-

174

tially because he is the first friend that he has ever lost, aside from his pal Coshi. Accepting death is never easy, especially when it is unexpected. What words of wisdom can we impart to Corey as he remembers the lifetime of his friend?

I sense his ache; after all, we forged a strong bond early on in our relationship. Wherever he goes, I go. I try to get him to play, even though I'm no young pup. He tries for my sake but is often overwhelmed. All I can do is stay by his side.

There is a Hebrew proverb that states, "Say not in grief 'he is no more' but live in thankfulness that he was." This proverb needs to be the message that we end with. Most lives are filled with regrets and grief. But remember, we must celebrate and enjoy what we have while we have it. Although I miss Puppy and Shrimp, I realize that life isn't forever. I have to be thankful for the time that I had with them. Sure, I wish that I had had more, but remembering the good times helps.

We shouldn't wait until tomorrow to tell others that we love or care for them. Do it now. Death causes pain and a sense of loss, but it doesn't mean our lives end. This may not seem fair, but this is the life we're given. The apple ripens only once. Joe Lewis suggested, "You only live once, but if you do it right, once is enough." Joe must have known Coshi, Puppy, and Shrimp because they knew how to live. It is their lifetimes that we remember, and we all rejoice in our time spent together.

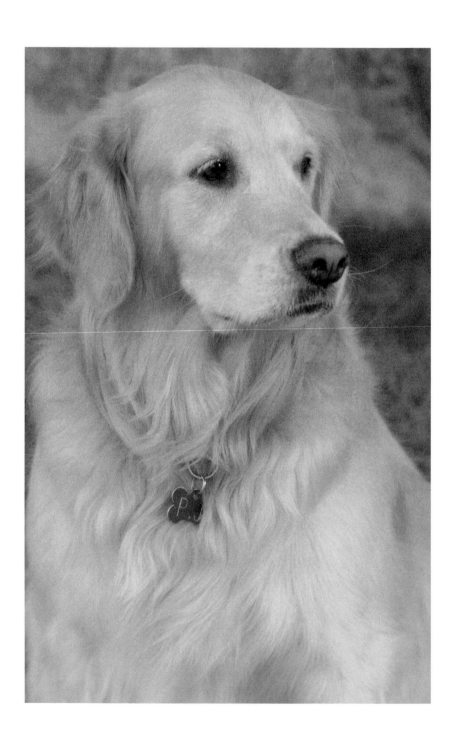

Serendipity Can Lead to Self-discovery

It has been almost seven years since Puppy left my side, but she has never left my heart. Wherever I am, I continue to have vivid memories of her. Like any strong relationship, ours was built on love, respect and my willingness to understand her needs. It is comforting to know that, although she has been gone for a while, she has left her mark upon so many people, especially me. I think of our days quite often, and how my afternoons next to her changed my life. Through our interactions, Puppy helped me become more compassionate and caring. I miss those days, even if I have my memories.

Ultimately, Puppy made her mark. Those who didn't live and work alongside her may not have noticed her inherent power. But I appreciated her benefits from the first day we met. I now realize, more than ever, that Puppy's spirit lives on within those she touched. She inspired by her example. Her ability to not give up on life and to persevere is a testimony of her tenacity. I am especially touched when past patients who knew Puppy continue to call and "relive" their experiences. Their interest in sharing how Puppy touched their hearts also keeps her spirit alive. Personally, Puppy revealed that wonderful things can happen with hard work and trust, but you must open your mind and heart to find them.

Although I've learned much through my observations, along with working and living with animals, I've also learned that life's lessons can come in many forms, such as a chance encounter. It's my sincerest wish that the stories and experiences I've shared in this book are helpful in guiding you toward a plan for living a more fulfilled life. But this discussion would not be complete without talking about serendipity, life's unplanned events, especially the seemingly small ones.

The term "serendipity" comes from a Persian fairy tale that explains the advantages of unplanned discoveries. So much of life can be serendipitous. We never know from day to day what may occur. Some outcomes in life may be planned, while others may occur just because we were there. These are the events that often are the richest life has to offer.

Having spent the past two decades in the company of animals, I've learned to prioritize what is important in life. Often we take things for granted or only appreciate people when they are no longer by our side. We miss the essence of why we are here if we follow this way of life. I remember the day we rescued Puppy. I used to think we were the ones that were sent to help her, but now I wonder if it was the other way around. For a girl who had such a rough start in life, she left the world with her head held high. She showed me that sometimes things that are worth having are worth working for. She also showed me that kindness, persistence, and forgiveness are more powerful traits than animosity, weakness, and blame. Throughout this book I've shared many stories that illustrate the power of the human spirit and how we can be more thoughtful and sensitive individuals. But as I've emphasized, it is also important to live each day as the very best person we can be, and animals are excellent teachers. It is fitting, then, to close this book with some parting advice, mottoes that I see my animals living every day.

Turn a Negative into a Positive

Sean, Puppy and I are about a block from home as we come upon a house with a rickety fence. As we pass, we hear barking. I look back and see a large rottweiler charging the fence. Just as I face forward I hear a loud crash. I look again and see the dog running toward us. My son and I are startled, but I encourage him to continue walking as we try to ignore what is coming from the rear. He is shaken and asks quietly, "Dad, are we going to get bitten?" The possibility is also crossing my mind, but I want to stay calm, for both our sakes. Just like in the movies, time slows and yet the dog is gaining on us.

Of the three of us taking the walk, Puppy remains the most confident. She wants to maintain her relaxed pace even though I am urging speed. She doesn't seem to notice or to be bothered by the dog running behind us. The rottweiler closes in enough for me to see his huge teeth sparkling in the sunlight. I quickly push Sean behind me and start to turn away. But unlike both of us, Puppy faces the large dog and immediately begins to wag her tail and then she lies down and is very still. This is her reaction to an impending attack? But, like Gandhi, Puppy has a positive response to defuse the hostility. I am sure she wants to protect, but she instinctively realizes that a harsh reaction will only escalate our situation. To my surprise, the dog doesn't attack Puppy, but begins to walk around her and sniff. Puppy holds her ground, continuing to wag her tail. What might have been a catastrophe is now being diffused.

——

After Puppy has averted a near disaster, we needed to take care of one other piece of business. Sean looked towards me and said, "Dad, we cannot leave the dog here. If we do, he could get lost or hurt." The dog was relaxed now, but resisted our efforts to have him follow us back to his house. Knowing that Puppy was dependable and obedient, I proceeded to take off her collar and leash and place it on the neck of our new friend. Now attached to a leash, we all walked him home and returned him to his backyard. Before leaving, we shared with him one of Puppy's dog biscuits. A tragedy was avoided, and we learned a major lesson: face a negative challenge with a positive solution. We were able to turn what we thought was an enemy into a friend. Puppy showed us the importance of accepting and being there for someone regardless of apparent dysfunctional behavior.

It was Puppy's relaxed nature that helped us understand that sometimes what looks bad might be nothing at all. More importantly, sometimes the unexpected can show us the unknown about others and ourselves. We can be so focused on fear that we never believe we can prevail. Sean and I still think of that day and the tremendous but unexpected lesson we learned.

Kindness Costs a Little Kibble but Goes a Long Way

In the chapter "Giving from the Hart," we met Sarah, who was going through a tremendous bout with anxiety and depression. The attention and care that Hart showered on Sarah helped her get through a tough time. When you think of it, Hart's acts of kindness helped Sarah relax and be more open to receiving help. It was through the gentleness of their relationship that Sarah developed the confidence to open up to the world around her. When we met for the very last time, I will never forget how Sarah embraced Hart. She held her and said, "You were the main reason I opened up." As Hart gazed into Sarah eyes, what were they both thinking? I only can surmise that it may have to do with the mutual kindness found in their relationship.

It's early in the morning and I stumble towards the front door to pick up the newspaper. I swing open the door and as I bend down I see Kitty sitting there with something in her mouth. As I bend closer she drops a dead mouse on the doormat. She sits back down and looks up at me with expectation, if not a hint of pride, as if to say, "See what I've done for you because I love you. And, by the way, thanks for letting me join your pack."

It's been over twenty years since we found Kitty, and even though she has long since passed away, I remember those gifts dropped on my doorstep. At the time we lived in a newly established neighborhood, and although it was urban, the area was remote and it had a country feel to it. We lived next to a large field and a short distance from numerous horse ranches. Kitty was either a feral cat, born in the wild, or abandoned. We adopted her, and our family, especially Sean and our first dog Goldie, quickly became great friends.

Kitty would join us on our family strolls through the neighborhood. Goldie would be by her side and it was breathtaking to watch them. They were kindred spirits, and the friendship between them was evident. Our love for Kitty grew, and she became an important part of our life. I truly believe that she knew that, hence the offerings.

Kindness comes wrapped in so many ways. Sure, we like gifts wrapped in tinsel and pretty paper, but acts of kindness can't be purchased. Kitty's actions were priceless and were genuine. Acts of kindness usually don't cost anything, but they can have a monumental impact.

Caring and Protecting Others Builds Self-confidence

When Hart joined our family, I knew that helping train her as a guide dog would be good for both of my boys. Sure, we wanted to be puppy raisers for the right reasons, but I have always known that caring and protecting others builds self-confidence. I learned to understand this when I began bringing Sasha, whom you read about in the chapter "Discoveries," to a social skills group for children who had learning disabilities. They loved taking care of her. Their acts of kindness in caring for her helped build their self-esteem. Giving to others allows us to recognize our own inner talents and our ability to be a contributor rather than a taker.

The same outcome occurred when we brought Hart into our family. She also was a tremendous teacher. She let the boys mentor and train her, but indirectly helped them grow and become more responsible. I especially remember the early mornings when Hart first came to our home. Corey was her caregiver and he would wake up in the early morning hours and take her outside to go to the bathroom. Even as tired as he was, he never was impatient. Once done, he ushered her back to his room and would fall quickly back to sleep. He became her knight in shining armor. She knew where to go for protection. Their relationship grew and Hart became an important dimension to Corey's early life.

Caring for others brings remarkable outcomes. Some say that such a human-animal relationship is a "magical" potion that can help us feel better. But there's no magic. It's the power of selflessly caring for another being that unlocks and strengthens our awareness of others and ourselves.

A colleague shared this next and final illustration, and it is an inspiring story about a client who managed to overcome the demons of her past, just by feeling needed. The client states: "I was consumed with sorrow and buried in the pain that I believed life had unfairly inflicted upon me. As a child, I was always on a mission: safety. I was constantly looking for safe places, safe people, and safe objects." She goes on to state that if safety could not be attained, she at least found a sense of peace through animals, but these, too, had to be safe.

Amber chose rabbits and while looking for a mate for her male, she discovered Zoë. Zoë and Stewart are Netherlands dwarf rabbits. However, when Zoë was four years old, her health deteriorated, and she depended on Amber even more. One day, while at one of the numerous vet visits, Zoë struggled out of the veterinarian's arms and jumped back into Amber's embrace. At first, Amber was startled and taken aback that Zoë was looking to her for protection. Later that night Amber realized what Zoë's action had communicated: "By simply being herself, Zoë's gifts to me were numerous."

"Zoë had a wonderful and regal way of making you think she was larger than she was. She had an air to her that just said, 'Look at me, I am special.' She moved with confidence, and although she wasn't huge, she was comfortable with herself. Zoë's self-confidence was an inspiration, especially to someone like me who had always felt small and vulnerable."

But not letting size dictate how we view ourselves is not the only reward Zoë gave her owner. Through Zoë's illness, Amber learned a lesson about giving to others. She realized that Zoë relied on her for safety and comfort just as much as, if not more than, she relied on Zoë. She stated, "If I could induce this feeling in Zoë, then my own 'safety' must be accessible. For over two decades I'd been searching for that sense of safety everywhere, not realizing I could find it within myself ."

As Amber was learning to love and care for Zoë and Stewart, she was also learning to love and care for herself. Through her love for the rabbits, Amber communicated that she could be trusted to give both comfort and safety to her pets. In turn, Zoë showed her trust in Amber. In caring for Zoë, she began to feel more comfortable with others, and a chink was made in Amber's self-imposed wall of seclusion from other humans. "How could I be scared and be afraid of taking care of myself, but at the same time be someone else's protector? Zoë helped me find myself and realize that I could care for others."

Caring for others has a direct link to healthier self-confidence. It is when we can look around and say that someone is looking towards us for security that we may begin to appreciate our own assets. For years, so many of my clients have relished the opportunity to take care of my animals. From caring for the birds to having an opportunity to dog-sit PJ or Magic, children realized that the animals were looking up to them. Steve once said of his time in taking care of Boomer, "Boomer never likes to feel caged, and that is why I make a point to get her out often." He realized that, just like himself, Boomer needed to feel more freedom, and he became the key to opening up her world. It was easy to transcend his experiences with Boomer and begin to discuss that he could be a caregiver rather than a care receiver. Although not a panacea, it was a beginning for him to see his value as a person.

Standing Up for Your Rights

Each day we need to practice taking charge and being an active participant in our own lives. When Cynthia first brought her cairn terrier, Darby, home to meet Belvedere, she thought the adjustment might be a bit rocky. To her and the family's surprise, though, Belvedere was welcoming, perhaps because he was the larger dog. Admittedly, they were an odd pair. Darby came up to the top of Belvedere's legs and Belvedere outweighed Darby by almost 70 pounds. However, Darby was not one to let size determine any outcome, especially when it came to what was his.

Darby had a favorite toy, a blue racquetball. He loved to have someone throw the ball for him to chase down and retrieve. From the start, Belvedere had never shown any interest in joining this activity and most often was content to lie in the shade and watch. Even if the ball rolled under his nose, he'd not move. But on one spring day he did. Belvedere grabbed the ball in his mouth, stood upright, and stared at Darby. For several moments Darby ran circles around Belvedere, all the while barking and nipping at his legs. When Belvedere failed to relinquish the ball, Darby chose his moment, jumped in Belvedere's face, and snatched the ball from his mouth.

I know it may be hard for some of us to be assertive, but it is a skill that we need to develop. We shouldn't sit on the sidelines when things happen of which we don't approve. If we witness an injustice, we need to speak up. Injustices can be mild or serious, personal or global. The point is that we must work on expressing how we feel about things. At times we will be uncomfortable, especially at first. But if we remain silent, we are too often left in a position where we feel neglected and unheard. Everyone's voice is deserving of attention, so make sure yours is heard.

Greet Your Loved Ones at the Door

As I slide the key into the front door, on the other side I hear claws clicking on tiles and dog tags jingling. I turn the key and open the door slowly so as not to hit any of the scrambling dogs, but through the opening comes an excited, sniffing muzzle. I step over the threshold and another cold nose touches my hand and tails are wagging wildly, banging against the floor, the wall, and me. As I close the door, I now can hear the birds calling out to me. They are all saying hello. To some this is chaos; to me this is home.

It always feels great when I come home and the dogs and birds are beside themselves with excitement and anticipation, waiting for their individual hello. What greater compliment can anyone give you than by saying or demonstrating how happy he or she is to see you? What can we learn from the simplicity of this action? I first became aware, truly aware, of this simple bonus after adopting Puppy. Before she arrived, I often came home to an empty house because my wife and sons were often out. Not until Puppy became a part of the family did I realize just how important a welcome-home can be. And not until I heard this story did I understand the devotion love can produce in an animal.

At the Shibuya Train Station in Tokyo there's a bronze statue of a little dog. This Akita, whose name was Hachiko, died in 1935 while waiting for his owner to return home on the evening train. This was a daily ritual for Professor Uyeno and Hachiko. Each morning the two would walk to the station and say their good-byes, and when the professor returned in the evening, there waiting would be his canine companion. No one knew what the little dog did during the intervening hours, but the regular passengers all knew that Hachiko would reappear at the appropriate time.

One day in 1925, Hachiko waited in vain. Professor Uyeno had died that day at the university. But Hachiko returned each day for ten years, patiently waiting. Sometimes he would sit in the same spot for several days, going without food and water. Upon his death, the small community erected the statue in honor of his love and devotion.

Being "greeted at the door" doesn't mean we must physically be waiting at the entrance, as do so many pets, such as Professor Uyeno's or mine. Rather, the thought behind this phrase simply means that we should take a few minutes to welcome home family members. If you're in the kitchen up to your elbows in dishwater, you can just call out a "hello," perhaps stating where you are. The idea is that we take the time to show we care about our loved ones. When a pet greets its owner, the animal is expressing not only a hello, but also sharing that the owner was missed, while also reaffirming a connection or bond.

While children may or may not be communicative upon arriving home from school, they will appreciate that you care enough to recognize their presence. Ironically, this is one of the first things that many children say they miss as they grow older and the family's schedule becomes more diverse. Coming home to an empty house, especially after a particularly good or disastrous day, can be a real letdown. Apathy, even at the smallest level, will quickly poison a relationship. Letting family members know they were missed helps build and maintain self-esteem. This small ritual also helps strengthen both the family unit and the bond between individual family members, showing love, appreciation, and devotion.

Love and Recognition Make a Difference in Everyone's Life

James says, "I was driving down Indian Hill Boulevard and saw you walking the dogs. It reminded me of when I was a kid, and we did the same thing. Is Puppy still alive? She was the greatest." I smile as I hear him talk endearingly about my old colleague, and for a moment she is alive once again in my mind. I tell him that she passed on over three years ago, and then introduce him to PJ and Hart. He comments on how much PJ looks like Puppy. It is neat to see PJ interact with the young man who had known Puppy. PJ quickly nudges herself close to him and, like Puppy, gets him to give her attention. Unfortunately, my schedule is tight this afternoon and we don't have too much time to catch up. I think, "What a glorious gift he's giving me by showing that I was an important part of his life." Although we haven't seen each other for many years, he has never forgotten our relationship. A simple visit for a quick "hello" has rekindled it all.

———

While rescuing animals who have had difficult lives, I never realized all the love that I would get back in return. The same holds true about my own work with children and their families. Some of the most meaningful rewards I have received in my career are the notes I get from parents and children telling me how much our relationship meant to them. Take James, for example. I found this young teen sitting in my waiting room one afternoon and didn't recognize him. I wasn't scheduled for a meeting, so his presence was even more baffling. He looked up when he saw me coming closer and said, "Do you know who I am, Doc?" I stumbled for a few moments, until I finally admitted that I didn't recognize him. I said, "Just tell me your first name, and I bet I will remember from there." I have always prided myself on remembering most of the children I have worked with, but as they age, their physical features change and they are not as easily recognizable. "My name is James," he quickly responded and waited to see if I did indeed remember him. Immediately all the memories of who he was came to mind: a fatherless boy, a loving grandmother as primary caregiver, his trouble staying focused, his difficulty getting along with others. But on this day I fully realized just how far he had come. After even a brief chat, I knew he'd become a warm and caring young man, one about to graduate from high school and attend college.

James's visit was more meaningful to me than most of the store-bought trinkets I receive. So how can we change our mindset to appreciate the little things in life? How can we appreciate what we have and elevate the value of our good fortunes? These are questions that each of us will find if we look deeper within ourselves. Some of us are so used to judging the material gifts we receive by size and cost that we ignore the simple ones. Yet in the long run, these non-material gifts, too often right in front of us, are priceless. A look, a touch, a soft breath against the back of my hand, are things I experience every day when I come home. How fortunate I am to have so much love waiting for me!

Digging for That Bone Is Hard Work, but Well Worth It

PJ and Magic love their squeaker toys, and as I sit here at my desk ready to end my day, I can hear one of them playing. In the next moment Magic joins me, still batting her toy. Then she begins biting, tugging, and wrenching it to and fro. As I watch, I'm reminded of a child digging to the bottom of Cracker Jacks or a cereal box to claim the promised prize. In turn, I am reminded of my mom and how angry she would get because I would cram my arm up to the elbow into the box. Cereal went everywhere, but it was all worthwhile. I look down at Magic just as she finally rips the toy open enough to claim her "prize," the squeaker mechanism. I go back to work, waiting for her to tire, standing by to make sure she doesn't swallow it. I'll wait because her hard work, determination, and joy of accomplishment should be rewarded.

Magic with her squeaker toy is like other dogs digging for bones. Dogs are tenacious and single-minded when searching for that bone, as is PJ or Magic in searching for that squeaker. Things worth having are worth working for. These are often words that we hear, especially at times when things aren't working out. But this should not be limited to only material objects, a fact that many of us may have forgotten. We need to remember that relationships and being the very best person that we can are really worth the hard work we put into them.

Many of you will remember Teddy, the nine-year-old golden highlighted in an earlier chapter, for her outward sensitivity towards a man who needed emotional support at a meeting about his child. But Teddy has many other talents, including being a beach aficionado and loving to play fetch in the water. Just watching her run on the beach and into water is exhilarating. I see the excitement and joy in her eyes and her actions. She's ready to play and is ready to play hard. A few months ago, PJ and Hart joined Teddy on a Sunday play date. Although my girls love the beach, there is no comparison to their friend. Teddy is so upbeat. She is jumping, waiting for the ball to be thrown into the ocean. Although she is nine, her playfulness reminds me of a much younger dog. Once the ball is released she races into the water and paddles out to retrieve her prize. The amazing part of this process is that her excitement in playing does not diminish over time. She is having a literal ball. What impresses me the most about "my fair lady" is that she never wants to give up, just like digging for that bone.

The other day I witnessed this type of event. The ball that was thrown out seemed to get lost in a shuffling wave and Teddy lost sight of where it landed. Not letting this detract her from her mission, she began to paddle and move through the water with grace. She didn't seem to get frustrated. On the contrary, her enthusiasm remained high. Eventually she rescued her prize and dashed back for the next round. She stayed the course and was rewarded.

Whether we're playing, learning, or advancing in our career, accomplishing goals is often all the more sweet if they aren't easy to attain. If we recognize that something or someone is important, we shouldn't back away from the challenge.

Years ago, I had the honor of meeting Bob Wieland. Bob lost his legs in Vietnam when he stepped on an 82 mm mortar. Throughout our conversation, I noticed that he didn't dwell on his past, on the war that took his legs and confined him to a wheelchair. He demonstrated his commitment to his new challenge by walking across America on his hands. His mantra, "It doesn't matter where you finish in the race of life, it only matters that you finish," inspires me throughout every race as well as in my daily life. One reason many of us don't accomplish a goal is because we're overly concerned with how others are doing or how they see us. Try not to worry about what or even how others think. It doesn't help the situation. Instead, compete against yourself and judge fairly and kindly.

Whatever you do, always remember that complaining won't help. Believe me, I've been there too. There are times that I have had to do things, and I did them despairingly. My attitude didn't help and it made doing what I had to do horrible. The same even happens with the dogs. Whenever bath time comes around, I have to almost drag the dogs in. It's funny to watch. Just hearing "bath time" makes them apprehensive. If they were human, I'd say they moan and groan. Hart hides under the bed, and PJ tries to run. On the other hand, Magic is enthralled with the entire process. Ironically, once we start the bath, Hart and PJ love our little ritual, which includes playfulness and cuddling. This is another good point to remember: what may at first appear unpleasant might just be a wonderful and fulfilling experience. We must realize that our dreams are at our fingertips, if we are determined to work for them. But a large part of this determination requires that we accept the occasional failure.

Learn How to Fall (or Fail)

I'm sitting, as I often do, watching Snowflake try to open her cage. She is amazing, a winged Houdini, albeit less graceful and successful. But this is part of the joy of watching her. Every time she slips, stumbles or falls from her perch, she simply gets back up and tries again. And although she rarely succeeds, she routinely tries to open the door. Snowflake is confident, determined, patient, and above all, not afraid of failure.

Tumbling and falling seem more readily acceptable in the animal world than in ours. Have you ever seen a squirrel racing across a tree branch, attempt to jump to another limb, only to crash-land on the ground, roll over, and race back up the tree? Why do we have the saying "cats always land on their feet"?

Avoiding a challenge can give us a false sense of success. To be truly successful we have to be willing to gamble and realize that falling is just part of life. We just have to learn to get right back up like that squirrel. Learning to fall is also a state of mind. We must be willing to accept that we might fall or fail. There is no shame in stumbling, either physically or emotionally, in some area of life. Failing to achieve a goal is not equivalent to failing life. Yet how many of us have been taught to think so? Learning to fall, or fail, gracefully takes practice and a willingness not to give up on either the goal or ourselves. There is no success without failure. Learning to make corrections makes us stronger and more confident.

Some Problems Require Unique Solutions

While I was in the United Kingdom a few years ago, I read about an unusual dilemma at the Battersea Dogs' Home. The morning staff was baffled as to how nine animals, over the course of several nights, were getting out of their kennels and indulging in a doggy midnight feast. Finally, the staff installed cameras to see what went on after hours. To their surprise, the culprit was a determined greyhound named Red the Lurch. When lights were out and the staff gone for the evening, Red slipped his slim muzzle through the bars, and using his teeth, he managed to open the latch. He proceeded to walk down the hallway and free the rest of the dogs on his corridor. Once everyone was out, they headed off to the kitchen.

Red's hard work paid off. He may have been locked up in a cage, but he was determined to break free. Red was identified as the ringleader and became a celebrity in Great Britain, with over four hundred families having applied to adopt him. The message is simple. Whenever we feel like retreating, muster the strength to push forward and rethink the plan. We only truly fail when our spirit is defeated.

Fortunately, our lives are built on many events, not only those that we fail or cannot accomplish. We should adjust our feelings of inadequacy and balance them so that we don't view ourselves as failures. We need to view failure as an event, not a person. These missed opportunities can be turned into lessons to learn from. They can help us understand what is needed to overcome these challenges in the future, or teach us what we may need to know to circumvent them. Perseverance means that we are determined and focused, as was Red the Lurch. He not only escaped his cage, but he also gained a freedom beyond his expectations, as well as a new loving family. But Red also freed the other dogs. His bravery and willingness to work around the obstacle not only made the escape possible, but also forged him into the leader of the pack.

Sniffing at All the Details Can Cause You to Wander off the Path

While walking my dogs, I've noticed just how often they are tempted off the path. A scent catches their attention or they feel the need to mark their territory. More often than not, they return quickly. But sometimes they become so occupied with a particular scent or they catch the eye of another dog, that I have a difficult time coaxing them back.

It is okay to stray off the path. It is important to appreciate the fact that slight detours are healthy. Leaving the path can lead us in a new direction that opens up new opportunities. However, sniffing at all the details can get us too far off the track and even lost. This can become more of a challenge, especially if we obsess on negative details. The negativity can detract from our momentum and get us further from our goal. We have to recognize that ruminating over our sorrows can sour the outcomes. We need to be determined in our efforts and point our vessel in the direction it needs to go. Using our internal compass with passion and optimism helps us steer the right course. With constant monitoring, even if we become a little sidetracked, we can sail in the right direction.

How many times a day do we let details and small incidents get in our way? With today's family going at life full tilt, things are bound to go wrong from time to time. Your Siamese will inevitably have a fit while you're in the shower, or your two-year-old will play "hide the keys" when you least expect it (on a practical note, duplicate keys are a must with toddlers in the house). Although such an event may require a shift in the schedule or a recalculation, the important thing to remember is that it is, after all, not life-threatening. Try to keep such occurrences in perspective; don't let them overpower you. Believe us, such events, given time, are the stuff of family legends.

Animals Learn How to Shake It Off

I'm standing in the backyard on a hot California afternoon holding my garden hose over my birds. They need a shower to help cool them and I'm enjoying watching as they first flap and then spread their wings to distribute the water. The sun glistens on the tiny, sparkling jewels of water droplets, but soon they begin flapping vigorously to remove the excess. Puppy wanders over to join me and I turn the hose on her. She stands patiently until she thinks she's soaked. But I'm on guard because her idea of what is enough is not consistent, and I must look for the signal or risk a soaking myself. There it is. She spreads her legs and looks up at me as if to say, "OK, here it comes," and then she begins to shake her golden fur.

Shaking off the water is part of the bathing process. The same should hold true with feelings that may be damaging to us. The other day, while I was at the dog park, a small Labrador kept digging. At first the owner was patient and tried to redirect the young pup. However, after about thirty minutes, he became very frustrated and when he caught her in the act, he reacted very sternly. The puppy seemed confused and also a little afraid. However, moments after being scolded, I saw the puppy run towards her companion, licking him tenderly. What is it about animals that make them more forgiving? Do they know something that we don't? Do they realize that holding on to anger can be one of the worst things we can do?

What is unique about my pets' actions is that these animals have learned it is necessary to shake off the excess weight. Many of us carry extra burdens that could and should be shaken off. One of the extra burdens some humans carry is anger, especially anger that evolves into a grudge. Animals don't seem to follow this belief system.

Every day I talk to families about letting go of anger and forgiving others. Their anger anchors them in a horrible place in their mind that unfortunately can be destructive to them. Holding on to anger or having a grudge towards others doesn't lead to solutions, but rather can intensify the anger within us and make it fester. Anger holds us down and often prevents us from working things through. We cannot expect to go through life unscathed by hurt, and most conflicts can be ended if each person is willing to listen, resolve, and then let it go. Prolonged anger and holding a grudge keeps us from moving in a productive and positive direction. When we do things to release our anger, the sole burden isn't on our shoulders. Releasing this enemy allows us to put our strength into fighting battles that are more meaningful.

Animals have disappointments, but they seem to let them go and give others a chance for redemption. A new day brings new beginnings. We should follow these actions. Yes, we can be disappointed, but rather than brooding, we need to learn to move on and take positive actions.

One positive action is to realize that some people aren't yet willing to change. If we find ourselves frequently at odds with a friend, then it may be time to reevaluate the relationship and assess why it is turning out the way it is. Sometimes people become less compatible as we grow, and we may need to move on. It may be hard at first, but it may be very necessary. Remember, new beginnings are okay; we have to have the courage to move on.

Another way to let go of the grudge is to evaluate just how important the issue is. If we can reassess the initial hurt, we often discover that in the long run, it's just not important. To begin the assessment, ask yourself the following questions: Why am I holding on to this anger? How is holding this grudge helping me? What could I be doing with all this energy if I directed it toward improving my life? Once we recognize that we can "shake it off," we may be more willing to release these anchors, and the result is that we will sail more freely and smoothly.

Be Happy for Others

Today is PJ's sixth birthday (where have all the years gone?), and it has been a special day for her both at home and at the office. She's received a few gifts, had special treats and has heard chants of "Happy Birthday" all day long. She especially loved the special meals we prepared for her breakfast and for dinner (the whole gang sharing, of course). When PJ was a puppy, she was put on a natural diet, and she loved her oatmeal, eggs and yogurt breakfast. This morning was not any different. She sat impatiently watching Nya prepare her treat. As always, she "hummed" while sitting in place.

I am so happy for her. I am quite certain she doesn't know why the day is so special, but she knows something is different. She has been pampered and loved it, and I couldn't be any happier. I've learned never to be afraid of sharing excitement for the accomplishments of others.

Reveling in the happiness and the successes of others is an action we should all follow. For example, each year at my university, a commencement luncheon is put on for a group of students with learning disabilities who have worked extremely hard to reach their milestone. They will not be the valedictorians of their class, but each of them demonstrates the tremendous commitment they have had to finish what they started.

At these yearly events I'm always brought to tears when I witness their joy and pride. I am happy for them and in some way my joy for them becomes uplifting for me. A simple motto I like is: "Be happy for others." We shouldn't envy what we don't have but, rather, celebrate what others receive. In return, they will be happy to share our joys and accomplishments.

The way to a more fulfilled and happier life is to open not only our minds, but also our hearts. We need to venture beyond our own concerns and comfort zone. This may be a challenge at first, so I suggest taking small steps, celebrating even the smallest moment, whether your's or someone else's. Believe us, the reward will be tenfold.

Animals Keep It Simple

The gang and I arrive home, but they don't act tired as they leap from the car and run past me and into the house. I enter to find them all waiting at the feeding area. Today Magic gulps her food down the fastest, runs from the room, only to return with her mouth loaded with toys and ready to play. It is a daily ritual, and although it has been repeated hundreds of times, I delight in her excitement and toss one of the toys she's dropped at my feet. She is home now and knows she can let her hair down, unfettered by the office "house" rules. As I toss another toy, I know she could do this all evening, maintaining the same energy and enthusiasm. To reciprocate, I exaggerate my enthusiasm because I cherish this bonding time. We've had this ritual for years, and by the time the evening is completed, everyone will have his/her share of roughhousing because for dogs this is not only a form of play but also a form of affection.

I know my life is richer every moment I am around them. As I have said so often, I went out to find a miracle in helping me work with children, and the miracle ended up finding me. Their tenacity for life is indeed their greatest attribute. There are no hidden agendas. For them, simplicity and a raw lust for life are the keys to contentment. They just engage and keep on going, and this is their strongest attribute. They appreciate every moment they have, and it's the daily ordinary moments they seem to enjoy the most. They wait at the door every day to go to work. It is part of their daily ritual, so going is expected. What is unexpected is how they relate with such endearing kindness and devotion. They really do follow the motto: Keep it simple.

As Puppy aged, she began to slow down significantly. Nevertheless, she didn't want to stay home. As I considered her semi-retirement, Hart was ready to take on the lead role as a therapy dog in my practice. She had been an understudy for a while and had the skills. The sad part was I didn't really consider Puppy's feelings. The first few days, as Hart and I prepared to leave, Puppy gazed at us with a look of hopelessness in her eyes. She loved her work, and didn't want to let it go. Why would she? The work place was a spot where she shared her love with others, but also where she also was showered with affection. Then a solution came to me. Puppy could go to the office, but on her own terms, work at her own pace. When awake, she'd contribute. If she were napping, I'd just give her best regards to the children. It was perfect, it was simple. Puppy retained her dignity and continued working almost to the day she died.

How often have we heard or said, "I wish I wasn't so busy"? When we think or say this, it's evidence that we've taken on too much; we've become victims to and slaves of our schedules.

Complex lives and/or complex solutions don't always lead to better lifestyles or improved responses to living. Why is it that I become somewhat envious when I hear the statement "the dog days of summer?" Is it because I visualize my dogs just relaxing and having a great time? Maybe their lives are simpler because they don't have the same competing demands, but maybe we can learn from this. We need to simplify rather than complicate; otherwise, we'll live a life full of regret rather than passion.

Life Is What You Make It: Always Has Been, Always Will Be

It is 10:00 a.m. in the morning. In a few more hours I will be off to work to spend another afternoon working with children alongside my extended family of colleagues. Every day is a new day, and I never know exactly what to expect. I am there for my patients, but I also realize that I am not alone in my work. I have the dogs and birds, as well as the fish and the lizards, to help me get closer to my clients. The animals share their love and devotion with my patients as much as Puppy did years ago, but like everything in life, each event is a little different and yet the fundamental lessons of life remain constant.

So many lessons for living can be learned from the animals and people that surround us. We just have to take the time to watch and listen. I've shared my discoveries because I believe we are all capable of making changes if only shown the way. Having "the gang" of animals as colleagues has made me rethink my personal and professional life. They have helped me clarify issues that I perhaps would have ignored. They have been my joy and shared my pain. They have shown me how to be gentle in times when I may have reacted more harshly. They have helped me set priorities to keep my life on the right course. I love what I do, but the animals have always supported my conviction "that you make a life, not a living." They have supported me in acknowledging what should be viewed as important. In essence, they have aided in my ability to demonstrate not only my humanity, but also that I am, after all, only human.

There is an old saying that states: "From every ending comes a new beginning." It seems apropos to apply this verse as we close our adventure. Life is filled with serendipitous twists and turns. We should not fear these opportunities but rather celebrate the unknown and discover what is right in front of us. Endings are sometimes hard to accept, but with each ending, we may find ourselves on the doorstep of a new start. All of my animal family members, however great or small, have made some contribution to my life.

From all of my afternoons with Puppy, I think I know how she'd close this book. From her I learned that life has many doors, and her advice would be: "Never be afraid! We only have to open one door to begin the journey to self-discovery."

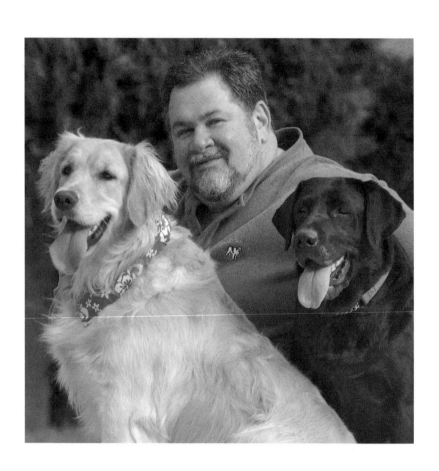

A Final Word

"The one absolutely unselfish friend that a man can have in this selfish world, the one that never deserts him, the one that never proves ungrateful or treacherous, is the dog. . . . He will kiss the hand that has no food to offer, he will lick the wounds and sores that come in encounter with the roughness of the world. He guards the sleep of his pauper master as if he were a prince."

—George Vest
Lawyer and U.S. Senator

Thanksgiving has just come and gone, and it was during this festive time that I decided to write these final words. The idea of writing *"Afternoons"* was given birth over four years. I believed then, as I do now, that the stories that you have read needed to be told and heard.

Early on as I began working on the book, I recall discussing the essence of these unique relationships with a few people. Although I piqued their interest, they were more fascinated when we discussed the "aha" outcomes. I guess that is expected, especially in a time when the media sensationalize the truly magnificent miracles sometimes found in human-animal relationships. These are outcomes so amazing that they take our breath away and touch our soul.

Personally, I am also still amazed by these media stories, but I also realize that most of life isn't composed of "aha" moments. Rather, most of our life experiences are the culmination of seemingly ordinary events that sometimes lead to terrific and powerful outcomes. These everyday actions are what we need to acknowledge and appreciate. Their impact shouldn't be underestimated. We have to respect the day-to-day contributions for what they are.

The relationships between animals and people shouldn't always be viewed for only the extraordinary outcomes, but rather the impact of an evolving relationship. If we do, we miss the brilliance of the process because we are too busy looking for the outcome. Miracles are found in the daily actions: the loving greetings, the tender caresses, the special times that make the bond a unique relationship. Hopefully *Afternoons* helped clarify this position.

Afternoons with Puppy was not only written to pay tribute to my therapy animals, but also for the many other therapy animals around the world who make a major difference. We need to acknowledge their efforts. Therapy animals' physical needs and welfare must be safeguarded so their quality of life continues to stay healthy.

Over the years, I have read hundreds of quotations celebrating the tender relationship between humans and dogs. Roger Caras's quotation has always intrigued me with his explanation of the importance of animals in our lives. He states that *"Dogs are not our whole life, but they make our lives whole."* His use of the word "wholeness" to describe how animals fulfill people's emotional needs is very appropriate. In essence, our connection with animals makes us feel complete. Just watch people play, walk, or just sit next to their beloved pets and you will personally witness that sense of wholeness. Our pop culture is also filled with many examples and artifacts that illustrate the importance of this bond. It is hard to walk through a store and not notice books, cards, and DVDs covered with attractive pictures of animals.

As we end, I hope you will consider the phrase *Afternoons with Puppy* as a metaphor for appreciating the inherent beauty found in the loving relationship with our beloved animal companions. The afternoons shared in this volume have been experienced by persons in need with trained therapy animals. Nevertheless, similar relationships are also established by millions around the world who have opened their hearts to their own animals. So to all who have these opportunities, enjoy your time and especially the afternoons. Not only will they enrich your life, but they will also feed your soul.

It's 11:50 a.m. and the "gang" is waiting; time for me to start another afternoon.

Additional References

Sources for quotations

Brownlee, Paula P. Keynote speaker and President Emerita of the Association of American Colleges and Universities. New York.

Caras, Roger. Animal rights activist and president of the ASPCA from 1991-99.

Hessler-Key, Mary. *From What Animals Teach Us: Love, Loyalty, Heroism, and Other Life Lessons from Our Pets.* Prima Publishing, Roseville, Calfornia, 2001.

Paschal Richardson, Isla. "To Those I Love".

Sucher, Jamie J. *Golden Retrievers Complete Owner's Manual.* Barron's Educational Series, New York, 2000.

Vest, George. Quote from Speech. Kansas City, 1870.

Williams, Ben. www.practical-pet-care.com/ezine. July, 2003.

References for Animal Assisted Therapy and Related Dog Resources

Becker, Marty. *Healing Power of Pets*, Hyperion Press, New York. 2003.

Chernack McElroy, Susan. *Animals as Teachers and Healers*, Ballantine

Books, New York, 1996.

Coren, Stanley. *How Dogs Think: Understanding the Canine Mind*, Free Press, New York, 2004.

Coren, Stanley. *Why Does My Dog Act That Way: The Complete Guide to Your Dog's Personality*, Free Press, New York, 2006.

Coren, Stanley. *Why We Love the Dogs We Do*, Free Press, New York, 2004.

Fine, Aubrey H. *Animal-Assisted Therapy: Theoretical Foundations and Guidelines for Practice*, Academic Press, San Diego, California, 2006.

McConnell, Patricia. *For the Love of a Dog: Understanding Emotions in You and Your Best Friend*, Ballantine Books, New York, 2006.

McConnell, Patricia. *The Other End of the Leash*, Ballantine Books, New York, 2002.

Mellonie, Bryan. *Lifetimes*, Bantam, New York, 1983.

Miller, Pat. *The Power of Positive Dog Training*, Wiley, New York, 2001.

<u>Organizations Supporting Animal Assisted Therapy</u>

American Kennel Club (AKC) Headquarters
260 Madison Ave
New York, NY 10016
(212) 696-8200
www.akc.org

Delta Society
875 12th Ave NE, Suite 101
Bellevue, WA 98005-2531
(425) 226-7357
(425) 235-1076 (Fax)
info@deltasociety.org

Therapy Dogs, Inc.
P.O. Box 20227
Cheyenne, WY 82003
(877) 843-7364
(307) 638-2079 (Fax)
www.therapydogs.com

Therapy Dogs International, Inc.
88 Bartley Road
Flanders, NJ 07836
(973) 252-9800
(973) 252-7171 (Fax)
tdi@gti.net
www.tdi-dog.org

North American Riding for the Handicapped Association (NARHA)
P.O. Box 33150
Denver, CO 80233
www.narha.org

American Humane Association
63 Inverness Drive East
Englewood, CO 80112
www.americanhumane.org

Pet Loss Hot Lines

The Iams Co. Pet Loss Support Hot Line:
888-332-7738

University of California, Davis:
800- 567-1526

University of Florida, Gainesville
800-798-9196

Contact PJ and Dr. Fine at their website

www.afternoonswithpuppy.com

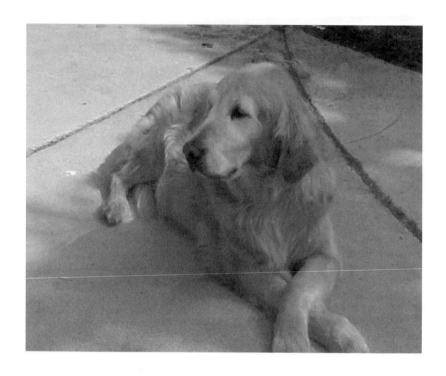

**In Memory of
"Puppy"
October, 2000**

All dogs have read Carl Rogers (Noted Humanistic Psychologist).
—Anonymous